your
best
life

The ultimate guide to creating the life you want

your best life

Don't just dream it – live it!

domonique bertolucci

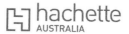

hachette
AUSTRALIA

Throughout this book you will come across this icon ⌐℮.
When you see it you can go to my website
www.domoniquebertolucci.com
for more information and additional exercises.

hachette
AUSTRALIA

Published in Australia and New Zealand in 2006
by Hodder Australia
(An imprint of Hachette Australia Pty Limited)
Level 17, 207 Kent Street, Sydney NSW 2000
www.hachette.com.au

Reprinted 2009

National Library of Australia
Cataloguing-in-Publication data

Bertolucci, Domonique.
    Your best life : the ultimate guide to creating the life you want

    ISBN 978 0 7336 2061 4.

    1. Life skills. 2. Personal coaching. I. Title.

646.7

Cover design by Ellie Exarchos
Text design by Christabella Designs and Bookhouse
Typesetting by Bookhouse, Sydney
Printed in Australia by Griffin Press, Adelaide
Author photo by Joanna Dye, www.JoannaDye.com

Hachette Australia's policy is to use papers
that are natural, renewable and recyclable products
and made from wood grown in sustainable forests.
The logging and manufacturing processes are expected
to conform to the environmental regulations
of the country of origin.

For my Mum and Dad

And for Paul
for everything, always

Contents

Preface   You only have one life, so it's important that you LOVE it!   1

Introduction   The three simple steps   7

Step 1   KNOW WHERE YOU WANT TO BE   15

Chapter 1   Discovering your dreams   17

Chapter 2   Understanding what matters   35

Chapter 3   Eliminating limiting beliefs and behaviours   57

Chapter 4   Creating a vision for your future   79

Step 2   KNOW WHAT YOU NEED TO DO   101

Chapter 5   Designing real and specific goals   103

Chapter 6   Developing unshakeable self-confidence   125

Chapter 7   Building a detailed plan of action   147

Chapter 8   Managing your resources   167

Step 3   DO IT!   189

Chapter 9   Developing amazing self-discipline and staying power   191

Chapter 10   Facing your fears and calling on your strengths   211

Chapter 11   Working through the tough times   235

Chapter 12   Celebrating your success   257

Author's Note   275

Acknowledgments   277

PREFACE

You only have one life, so it's important that you LOVE it!

Today is the first day of the rest of your life — what kind of life do you want it to be?

Have you ever wondered why life seems easy for some people? They're confident and in control, they have great jobs, happy relationships and love life. Why do these people radiate success? How did they create such dream lives? What is their secret?

The truth is, there is no secret. They are focused on what they need to do and who they need to become to create their dream life. They are following some simple steps and are committed to being the best they can be.

By working out what you want from life, what you need to do and who you need to become to make it happen, then simply going ahead and doing it, you too can create your dream life.

I have written this book to inspire, encourage and motivate you to continually be the best you can be. By maintaining this focus, you too will begin to create the kind of life you have been dreaming of – one that is filled with success and happiness.

If you have a goal, however big or small, you really can achieve it. You might find it hard work and sometimes you might want to give up, but if you persevere, you can live the life you've always dreamed of.

I have always been a positive, motivated person, but there was a time when I didn't feel like I was living my best life. Things were certainly going well and my life looked good on paper: a former model, a well-paid corporate job, a nice house, car and boyfriend. But I felt like I was living someone else's life; my success felt two-dimensional.

I found a personal coach and began to work out what 'success' really meant to me, and how I wanted my life to be. I remembered what my dreams had been and came up with some new ones too. I set about creating the kind of life that somewhere deep inside I knew I had been dreaming about.

It wasn't always easy; there were times when I wanted to give up or take an easier path. But I didn't give up. Every day I concentrated on being the best I could be, and worked hard towards creating a life that felt successful and satisfying.

I went from earning good money in a full-time job to six-figure short-term contracts. I worked for the companies of my choice and the hours I wanted and took the holidays I needed.

I left my boyfriend and met my soul mate. I moved cities and at times it felt like I moved mountains. I lost weight, felt great and knew that I was finally living my best life.

After ten years in the corporate world I took the lessons I had learnt and my personal experiences and qualified as a professional coach. My new business grew quickly and before long I had clients throughout Australia, the UK and the USA.

My next dream was to write this book so I could share what I've learned over the years – to inspire you to discover where you want to be, what you need to do and how to go about doing it. I want you to be able to create the life of your dreams too.

As a coach I have the wonderful opportunity of learning so much from my clients. Of course I've heard it on good authority that most of them learn a few things from me too! This book gives me a chance to share all of this with you.

One of the most important lessons I have learnt is the importance of pursuing *real* success – success that is meaningful and fulfilling.

Real success means success that is meaningful and fulfilling for you.

Very few paths in life are right or wrong, so it's important that you make choices that are right for you. Don't waste your energy pursuing someone else's dreams for your life. Don't do what you think you should be doing or chase ideals you think you should be chasing – real success is rarely just about houses, cars and boats. Instead discover what really matters to you, and design your success based on your own dreams, values and ideals.

I have made several choices that other people might have seen as the wrong ones: I left a man who loved me, I turned down a promotion and I walked away from the pinnacle of corporate success to start a new career in a new country.

Through it all, my life has been filled with friendship, variety, challenge, happiness and love. That is what *real* success means to me, and throughout this book I will show you how to discover what real success means to you.

My work is all about supporting people as they strive to be the best they can be – in both their personal and professional lives. I work with entrepreneurs, managers, executives, home-makers and students and I find that it doesn't matter what your age or stage in life – if you want to find *real* success and happiness, the same basic principles apply.

As you read this book and complete the exercises, you will start the journey of creating your own dream life. You will develop a strong and positive mindset and learn how to create a plan of action. You will discover strengths you never knew you had, and develop the skills you need to use those strengths to your advantage. You will gain new insight into who you are, what you want and what you need to do to make it all happen.

Although the first time you read this book you will probably benefit most by reading it from cover to cover, I hope that you will continue to refer to it, chapter by chapter, or specific chapters at different times, over the course of your life as your dreams grow and evolve and as you discover new ones.

That is my goal – to write a book that will become your trusted friend, guide and your very own coach.

INTRODUCTION
THE THREE SIMPLE STEPS

Looking back over both my corporate career and my coaching business, I've discovered that the key to achieving any goal in life can be broken into three steps:

> know **where** you want to be
> know **what** you need to do
> and **do** it!

These steps aren't rocket science; they're really quite simple. But at the same time they are also very powerful. Once you understand these steps there is absolutely nothing holding you back from achieving any goal you choose.

In this book I look at each step in detail. Within each step the text is divided into chapters that contain a wealth of information, not just to help you work out what you want, but also to create the skills you will need to help you go out and get it.

You might already know that one of the most important starting points is the right frame of mind – a positive mental attitude. But it takes more than just positivity to go after what you have been dreaming of.

Here is a summary of what you will learn:

STEP 1: KNOW WHERE YOU WANT TO BE

The first step towards creating the life of your dreams is to find out exactly what you want. Too many people chase after what they think is their dream without thinking it through, only to find that they are left cold and empty when they get there.

Step 1 of this book will help you to make sure that the dreams you are working towards are not only right for you but that achieving them will bring you happiness and fulfilment.

In *Chapter 1 Discovering your dreams* you will learn how to capture your dreams. Get back in touch with the lost art of daydreaming and start imagining a more inspiring and satisfying life. What would your life be like if you lived every day to your full potential? This is your chance to be bold. Later in the book you will find out how to make your goals achievable, but for now it's your turn to dream and dream *big*!

Chapter 2 Understanding what matters looks at what is important in life – to you. One of the biggest causes of frustration, stress and a sense of depression is living a life that is inconsistent with your values. But what are your values? You'll discover what makes you tick and what you can happily live without.

Chapter 3 Eliminating limiting beliefs and behaviours – time to do some more work on the most important element in your plan: *you!* This chapter shows you how to examine your thought processes and eradicate your limiting beliefs the things that stop you from making progress. It also looks at unproductive habits and behaviours and shows you how to put in place new ones to help you on the path to your dreams.

Chapter 4 Creating a vision for your future is about fine-tuning your vision working out what you really want and understanding what you are willing to do to get it. Clarify in your mind what you don't want and what you are not willing to compromise or sacrifice to achieve your dreams.

STEP 2: KNOW WHAT YOU NEED TO DO

Having a dream is not going to get you very far if you don't know precisely what you need to do to achieve it. In **Step 2** you will work out what you need to do and, importantly, who you need to become to create the life of your dreams.

In *Chapter 5 Designing real and specific goals* you will learn how to create SMART – Specific, Measurable, Attractive, Realistic, Time-based – goals and how to make these goals personal and meaningful.

You might even find that your goals are easier to achieve than you think!

Sometimes the hardest thing about achieving your dreams is the work you need to do on the inside: becoming the person you need to be to live your best life. There might be times when you feel like you can't do it, that perhaps you're not good enough. In *Chapter 6 Developing unshakeable self-confidence*, not only will you learn how to build your confidence and self-esteem, you will develop the strength and courage to pick yourself up and dust yourself off if things don't go your way.

Chapter 7 Building a detailed plan of action helps you create a step-by-step plan for achieving your goals. This plan will become your blueprint for success, providing you with affirmations to encourage and inspire your progress. You will also identify some key points at which you will well and truly deserve to celebrate your success!

Chapter 8 Managing your resources looks at some of the factors that can stop you from achieving your goals: how you manage time, money, health and fitness, sleep and energy, plus other resources you can call on when building your plan, including help from a friend or loved one, expert advice or creating your own support network.

STEP 3: DO IT!

Without action, there will be no results – **Step 3** is all about *doing it*. You know what you want and you have a plan to achieve it.

In *Chapter 9 Developing amazing self-discipline and staying power* you will learn how to create positive new habits and a mindset in which you can achieve anything that you set out to do.

Going after your dreams can be really scary. *Chapter 10 Facing your fears and calling on your strengths* advises you on facing your fears. It also helps you examine your strengths and look at how you can use them to your advantage along the way.

I'd love to tell you that the road to your dreams is going to be easy, but we all know that there are times in life when we feel like giving up. Sometimes those obstacles might be imagined, but other times they will be very real. *Chapter 11 Working through the tough times* focuses on meeting your challenges head on and staying on track.

Chapter 12 Celebrating your success: saving the best for last, the final chapter is about celebrating success and, equally as important, acknowledging all your successes along the way. After all, living your best life is not just a destination, it's a journey!

MAKING THE MOST OF THIS BOOK

1. Do the exercises

Life is for living, not skimming! The exercises I have set out for you are the same as those I ask my clients to complete. If you breeze through the chapters without setting aside time to work through the exercises the only person you will be short-changing is yourself.

2. Use a file or journal

Keep all your notes and exercises in one place. Some people like the process of physically writing things down, others prefer to type (I know that at least when I type I have half a chance of keeping up with my thoughts!), but whatever your preference, the most important thing is that you capture your thoughts, dreams and ideas in one place. By the end of this book you will have been on an incredible journey of self-discovery, you will have learnt so much about yourself and about the steps you need to take to achieve the most fulfilling and satisfying life. This journal will be your record of that journey.

3. Visit the website

I have created a special section on my website just for readers of this book. So make sure you visit www.domoniquebertolucci.com/yourbestlife where you will find a range of *free* resources including worksheets, tools, templates and extra tips, all designed to give you extra support as you begin to create the life of your dreams.

Whenever you see this icon there will also be a tool or template specifically created to help you complete that exercise.

4. Be honest

It's only by being completely honest with yourself that you will be able to achieve your true potential. Acknowledge your private and innermost thoughts. Be proud of your dreams and desires. You only get one life, and this is your chance to make sure that you really do LOVE it!

Step 1

KNOW WHERE YOU WANT TO BE

CHAPTER 1
Discovering your dreams

The first and most important step in creating the life of your dreams is to know what those dreams are. Most people are so busy living their everyday life that they don't know where to begin.

When you were a child you probably spent hours and hours daydreaming and enjoying make-believe adventures — maybe you were a princess in a faraway castle, an adventurer on the high seas or in the darkest jungle. In my favourite adventure I was Wonder Woman saving the world from evil with my magic lasso and bullet-proof bracelets. Saving the world with aluminium bracelets wasn't likely, but the point is, it didn't matter. When we were young, we didn't think twice about suspending reality and moving into a world where anything was possible and everything turned out exactly how we wanted it to.

Somewhere along the way, most of us were told to get our head out of the clouds, to stop being unrealistic, and to become responsible, sensible adults. We sat for exams, got jobs, houses, cars, credit cards and got on with it. Not only did many of us lose sight of our dreams; over time, we forgot how to dream altogether.

By reading this chapter, not only will you learn how to dream again, you will capture and explore your wildest dreams and will be ready to begin creating your own reality.

FINDING THE TIME TO DREAM

They may no longer be filled with superheroes and death-defying adventures, but do you know what is in your dreams today? One of the great casualties of modern life is that people no longer have enough spare time to think, let alone dream. Lives are filled with mobile telephones, emails, gym classes, late nights, early starts, and a whole range of family and relationship commitments. Technology means you are simply never on your own anymore. Even quiet times can be interrupted by a call on your mobile or filled with music from your iPod.

If you are to begin creating the life of your dreams then your first priority must be finding the time to dream. If like most people in the 21st century you lead a busy life, finding the time and space to dream can be quite a challenge, but one that you need to commit to if you want to fill your life with *real* success and happiness.

Start by finding some quality 'me' time each and every day. Think of the things that you enjoy doing. Allow yourself time each day to do one thing that really will be just for you. It could be a luxury like a massage, or it might be as simple as taking a 20-minute coffee break with your favourite book or magazine.

**Allow yourself time each day
to do one thing that really is just for you.**

Finding 'me time' doesn't have to result in a major shift in your routine or create a sense of 'one more thing that I have to do today'. It's just about taking the time to get back in touch with *you*. You might decide to create some 'me' time by walking all or part of the way to work each day or you could even start using your gym membership!

To gain the full benefit of your 'me' time, you need to ensure that at least some of it is spent in total silence. While music may be a pleasure for some people, for many it is just one more distraction. Turn off the TV or radio and simply relax in your own company. You might even want to learn to meditate or take a relaxation class, but most importantly, just breathe and enjoy being you.

One of the biggest challenges in finding some time to yourself can be all the commitments you have to others – husbands, wives, brothers, sisters, children, friends and co-workers – but with some careful planning, not only can you create your own 'me' time, you can also support others in finding theirs too.

When you do find yourself somewhere miles away, in the depths of a daydream, *don't* tell yourself to snap out of it. Instead, enjoy the moment and try to see where that dream takes you – of course this advice comes with a warning if driving a car or using machinery!

Although daydreams are often a mixed-up concoction of thoughts and ideas, examining them can lead to a better understanding of who you are and what you really want out of life. The best way to do this is to keep a journal. Make a note of your thoughts, feelings and dreams. Don't censor yourself, just write down whatever comes to mind. A journal is a private document; you never have to show it to anyone. But just like your daydreams, capturing your innermost thoughts and feelings on paper, and taking time to examine them, can teach you a lot about yourself. By taking note of your thoughts and feelings you might find the key to your dreams.

Your dreams are your own. Don't feel embarrassed or try to hide them. Simply enjoy exploring them for the secrets they hold.

Exercise

Think back over all the things you wanted to do with your life when you were younger. A good place to start is the ages between six and sixteen. It is likely that during these years, before college, work and 'real life' set in, you were bold in your fantasies about the future.

Make a note of all the ideas you can remember having. Just like a brainstorming exercise, this doesn't need to be in any order or make much sense to anyone but you. When you have captured everything you can remember, look back over your notes and see what patterns, themes and discoveries emerge.

When I did this exercise, one of the things I discovered was that all my childhood dreams had involved being in the public eye in some way… Wonder Woman, a movie star, a barrister, and even the prime minister for a brief moment! Look back at your dreams and discover the secrets they hold for you.

ENJOY THE LIFE YOU HAVE TODAY

It is easy to think about all the things you would like to change about yourself or your life. You might want to lose weight, get a better job, find a new partner or leave the one you're with. But it's important that all this thinking about the future does not stop you from enjoying your life as much as you possibly can today.

Just because there are aspects of your life you would like to change as you work towards creating your dream, it doesn't mean your life today is a disaster. Make a point of seeing the positive in every experience and start celebrating the good things about your life right now.

That 'life is a journey and not a destination' might be a cliché, but that doesn't mean it isn't true. A fundamental part of finding and living your *best life* is to enjoy it, each and every step of the way.

Exercise

It's important to acknowledge what is good in your life, and what you would like to change. Start by listing six things you value and appreciate about yourself and three things you would like to change, then six things you value and appreciate about your life and three things you would like to change.

Most people find it much easier to fill the list of changes they would like to make than the list of things they are happy with. Creating the right balance between striving for the future and enjoying today is important, so this is why for every item you add to the 'change' list, I have asked you to add two to the 'value and appreciate' list.

IF YOU WANT TO ACHIEVE IT, YOU NEED TO BE ABLE TO SEE IT

By now you probably have a good list of things you would like to change about your life. But do you know exactly what you would like these changes to be? If I gave you a magic wand or offered you a genie in a bottle, would you know what to wish for? It's one thing to know that you want changes, and quite another to know what you would like those changes to be.

So many people strive for change in their lives without knowing what they actually want and end up creating a constant sense of loss and disappointment. They might be successful but they don't feel satisfied. If you are to start living your best life, not only do you need to acknowledge all the things you value, appreciate and enjoy about your life, you also need to know precisely what you would like to improve or enhance in your life.

From now on, when you find yourself thinking that your life could be better, take the time to discover exactly what you would like to change and what would need to be different. If you don't take time to answer these questions then all you are doing is whingeing – and that's hardly constructive, is it!

START WITH A PERFECT WORLD

You might have heard the expression 'you create your own reality'. I certainly believe it's true. If you are going to begin creating your own reality, start by imagining that the world is a perfect place.

Yes, I know – life is not perfect. 'Reality' is filled with inconveniences and constraints, obligations and disappointments, but I believe that the phrase 'you're not being realistic' is toxic. It poisons people's ideas, hopes and dreams, snuffing them out before they can be fully explored. No, the original idea might not be possible, but if you don't explore it fully, how will you know how much could in fact become your reality?

In my professional experience, when you ask people what they believe *is* realistic, their expectations are far too narrow. Not only do they allow for inevitable constraints, they actually create pessimistic expectations of the potential outcome.

I want you to set reality aside for the moment and begin the vision of your dream life from the point of view of a perfect world. This allows you to imagine what life would be like if things went 100 per cent your way, 100 per cent of the time. It allows you to begin to enjoy thinking about things you once might not have believed possible.

Don't worry, I'm not suggesting that you become delusional, I'm just suggesting that the perfect world vantage point is the best possible starting point. Once you begin capturing (in your journal!) your dreams, ideas and fantasies you will have plenty of time to explore how to create your new reality. You will find that starting with the perfect world allows your dreams to be bigger and bolder than they might otherwise have been.

George's story

George is the managing director of a successful company. He sought coaching to work on his communication and motivation skills – he wanted to improve his communication with some new employees he had acquired as a result of a merger.

During our coaching sessions it became apparent that although George was successful and happy with the status quo, he also

(continued)

harboured a secret dream of taking a sabbatical in Europe. When I challenged him to explore his dreams further he realised that he had always wanted to own an award-winning vineyard, but had thought that this was far-fetched and unrealistic.

George used our coaching sessions to build on his already substantial management and leadership skills, paying particular attention to communicating with employees who came from a different background and culture to his own. Staff motivation increased and George was able to relax about the new employees fitting in.

Early in the coaching process George discovered that a sabbatical in Europe, after 20 years of service, was not actually unreasonable. It was achievable with a bit of careful planning and forethought. He has now set the date for his sabbatical and is focusing on both a development plan for existing staff and a recruitment initiative to ensure that his business runs smoothly in his absence.

George has also realised that the idea of a vineyard does not have to be a pipe dream and he is investigating the idea to find out if it is something he would really like to do, or just an idealised vision. He has set a provisional goal of owning and managing this new venture in ten years' time – when he retires from his current role. Should his research provide positive answers, he wants to make sure he is already on track.

THE DIFFERENCE BETWEEN DREAMS AND FANTASIES

You really can have anything you want in life, if you are willing to work for it. However, just because you find an idea desirable, it doesn't mean you would enjoy it, with all its consequences, if it was part of your everyday life.

You really can have anything you want in life, if you are willing to work for it.

In George's perfect world, he didn't have one special woman in his life. In his perfect world he actually had a glamorous woman in every port, to entertain him as he enjoyed his world travels. But in reality, not only was George happily married, he really wanted it to stay that way!

Therein lies the beauty of the perfect-world approach. It allows you to fully explore your imaginary life, then decide which bits of it you would like to incorporate into reality and which bits you are happy to keep as fantasies.

Explore your perfect world and determine which elements are dreams – things you really would like to have at some point in your life – and which elements are fantasies – yes, you'd have them if that genie did come along, but if the genie doesn't appear then you can definitely live without them.

Another way to think of it is to consider the level of regret you'd feel if you never experienced elements of your perfect world. What can you live without and what would leave you on your deathbed with questions of 'what if'?

Just because you don't need the full experience of something in your life doesn't mean that you can't enjoy elements of it. You might decide you don't actually need to be an Academy-Award®-winning actress, but that doesn't mean that joining your local theatre group won't be a rewarding and enriching experience. Having a fantasy isn't unhealthy, as long as you recognise it for what it is.

When you've finished the next exercise you will begin to see what your dream life might actually look like.

Exercise

Using the perfect-world exercise as your starting point, make a list of the dreams you would like to see become a part of your reality. Although I don't want you to worry about being 100 per cent 'realistic' yet, make sure you leave out all the elements that really are just fantasies.

Describe your dream life in as much detail as possible. You might find it helpful to group your thoughts under the following headings: health and fitness, financial security, relationships, family and friends, social life, recreation time, working life, holidays, and so on. You could write this as a list, or if you are feeling creative you could write a story about a day in your dream life.

THE POWER OF POSITIVITY

A client once asked me, 'If I do all of this, am I not just setting myself up for a big disappointment? Won't I just be depressed when my dreams don't come true?'

It was a valid question, but one that was based on her own negative outlook and a fear of failure. If you find yourself questioning things in this way, remind yourself that you are a unique and special human being, and that you really do deserve to live your very best life.

I'm not promising that every single one of your dreams will become a reality, but if you know what your dreams are, you will have a much better chance of creating a reality that includes them.

Creating the life of your dreams might not always be easy, but you do need to believe it is possible. You need to believe that you can make it happen and, most importantly, that you really do deserve it.

START LIVING YOUR DREAM LIFE – RIGHT NOW

As the saying goes, Rome wasn't built in a day, and creating the life of your dreams won't be an overnight task either. It takes time to make changes in your life, for your hard work to show results and dreams to become reality.

One of the best ways to accelerate the process is to look at the essence of your dreams and start investigating ways to incorporate that essence into your everyday life. Perhaps you long to live in Paris? Why not join the Alliance Française and start absorbing the French language and culture. Maybe you want to lose weight and completely change your image? Start with a new hair style and colour. You want to be a best-selling author? Start attending book readings and 'meet the author' evenings.

> **It takes time to make changes in your life, for your hard work to show results and dreams to become reality.**

For each and every one of your dreams there will be simple steps you can take to make the essence of that dream a part of your everyday life. The more often you get to enjoy dreams right now, the easier it will be to work towards bringing them to fruition.

You might find it takes a little creative thinking, but with all the practice you have had imagining what your dream life might be like, I am sure you're up to the task!

Annabel's story

Growing up, Annabel had dreamed of being an actor or movie star. She loved drama and had a starring role in all her high school productions. An intelligent teenager, she was encouraged to put this intellect to 'good use' and go to university. She decided to study law as she was fascinated by the glamorous characters on the television show *LA Law*.

Now in her late thirties and living in New York, the part Annabel enjoyed most about her work as a lawyer was when she was in court addressing the jury with her closing arguments. She secretly felt like the lead actor in a Shakespearean tragedy. As much as she enjoyed this aspect of her job, the rest of her work left her cold. After the intense high of being in a courtroom, win or lose, Annabel always came away feeling a little down.

She came to see me because she couldn't help feeling that something was missing from her life. She wondered what she might have been doing if she hadn't chosen this path, or whether she had wasted the opportunities of her youth. One thing she did know was that somewhere along the way she had lost sight of her dreams.

(continued)

I encouraged Annabel to stop thinking about the past and to focus on her future. What did she want it to look like? When she thought about her dream life, she was always on stage, enjoying the applause of her audience or accepting an award for best actress. She was always surrounded by creative people who were passionate about theatre, film and the arts.

She decided it was time to bring more of her dreams into her everyday life. She posted an ad in her law society magazine, looking for other lawyers who might be interested in forming an amateur theatre troupe. She was inundated with responses! It seemed that a lot of lawyers were frustrated performers.

When Annabel began rehearsing for what was her first performance since high school, she felt truly alive. It didn't matter that she wasn't getting paid; her dreams hadn't been about the money, they had been about performing.

Enlivened by this change in her life, she decided it was time for a career change too. Although she still enjoyed the income and security of life as a lawyer, she found a job in a firm that specialised in entertainment law. Annabel was determined that she would spend her working time surrounded by people who shared her passions.

DON'T BE AFRAID OF THE FUTURE

They say there are only two things in life to be afraid of – success and failure. Discovering your dreams can be quite overwhelming and may leave you with conflicting emotions. You are imagining how much your life might change if you were to begin living your best life, but the process of imagining this change can be quite confronting.

One of the best things about not having a magic wand or a genie is that you can work on creating your dreams over time. As they draw closer, you might find that they need adjusting or that other people might need to adjust to you.

Your dreams are yours. You and only you can decide how much or how little of them you need in your life.

Exercise

Make a list of your biggest fears. This might be a mix of both success- and failure-based fears. Next to each fear I want you to begin formulating your strategy for addressing it. Don't worry about describing your fears in detail – that will only reinforce them – just make sure you capture them all.

Perhaps there is something specific you can do to alleviate your fear, or maybe you simply need to accept it and forge ahead, without letting it hold you back in any way.

Overcoming your fears is discussed in detail in Chapter 9, but for now I just want you to get them out of your heart and onto paper.

If at any time you decide that you don't like the consequences of your dream, or that in fact it was just a fantasy, you are free to change your mind. Acknowledge your fears and look at them as an opportunity to learn more about yourself. Begin seeing your fears as challenges along your journey, not barriers preventing you from getting started.

BECAUSE YOU'RE WORTH IT!

You really are worth it. There is absolutely no reason why, if you are willing to work hard, you can't fill your life with all the success and happiness you desire. You really can live the life you've always dreamed of!

After completing the exercises in this chapter you should have a much clearer idea of what the life of your dreams looks like – the first and most important step in achieving it.

KEY LESSONS – DISCOVERING YOUR DREAMS

1. Find time to dream – it will be a valuable investment in your future.

2. If you want to create the life of your dreams, you need to acknowledge all the positive things about your present life. Make sure you are enjoying today, not just striving for tomorrow.

3. When you think about changing your life, be as specific as possible about what and how you would like it to change.

4. Remember, you create your own reality, so start with a perfect world and work back from there.

5. There is a big difference between dreams and fantasies. Fantasies are perfectly healthy, as long as you recognise them for what they are.

6. To achieve your dream life, you need a positive mental attitude. You have to believe that not only can you achieve it, you really do deserve it.

7. Find a way to include your dreams in your reality. The more often you get to enjoy dreams now, the easier it will be to work towards bringing them to fruition.

8. Don't be afraid of your dreams – you deserve to live your best life!

CHAPTER 2
Understanding what matters

Before you can create the life of your dreams – one that is fulfilling in every way – you need to know what matters most to you. What is important in your life, and what can you happily live without?

Some people think they already know the answer to this question and it usually includes family, friends, love, money and health. But I'm going to ask you to dig a little deeper and explore your *core values*. When you have uncovered your core values, not only will you find out exactly what it is about family, friends, love, money or health that is most important to you, you will also have a clear understanding of why.

Your values can evolve and change over the years. When I was younger, 'fun and excitement' held an important place on my list of values. While enjoying myself is still very important to me, this core value has now been replaced by 'stimulation and enjoyment'. Although they sound similar, for me they're quite different.

That brings me to the essence of why defining your values is so worthwhile. It's about working out what matters most to *you* and, importantly, having a deep understanding of *why* it matters.

If you are going to create your dream life, you need to know what *your* core values are. To do this you need to set them apart from the values of your environment and your upbringing and decide what it is that you, an intelligent, thinking, feeling adult, cherish most in your life.

Different words mean different things to different people. To one person, 'freedom' might mean having nothing that ties you down; to another, it might mean having everything money can buy. When you have worked out what matters most to you, you will be able to create a foundation for a future that is exciting, fulfilling and everything you have always dreamed of.

WHAT ARE VALUES AND WHY ARE THEY IMPORTANT?

Your values are the DNA of your soul. They are the key to what matters most to you in the world. Each of us has our own unique combination of values. They form part of our character and heavily influence the choices we make throughout life.

Your values are the DNA of your soul.

Put simply, your values are the aspects of your life that are of most *value* to you. Although just a series of words, your values hold a powerful insight into who you are, and how you are distinct from every other person on this planet.

Having a clear understanding of your values makes it easier to set goals, make decisions and create a fulfilling future. When you are living a life that is in alignment with your values, you will feel satisfied and content.

Successful and still not satisfied?

Most 'success' looks good on paper, but if what you are working towards is not in alignment with your values, your achievements may leave you feeling hollow and unfulfilled. If you want to be truly satisfied in life, you need to make sure that the choices you make and the success you strive for directly support one or more of your values. If the choices you make do not support your values, you can be left feeling annoyed, angry or lost, despite the success everyone else might think you have.

Alex's story

Alex is an entrepreneur in his early forties who has been responsible for several successful technology company start-ups. He has never been afraid of working hard and going after what he wants. He came to see me because, for all his professional and commercial success, he felt something was missing in his life. Not only was he single, he felt he didn't know who his good friends were anymore. He often felt lonely, even when he was with a group of people.

(continued)

Despite his considerable wealth, Alex was not a materialistic person. He was actively involved in several charities and community projects, and did not like flashy cars and clothes. During his first coaching session, before we even began to discuss values, he told me, 'Money just doesn't matter to me.'

Alex and I spent one of our early coaching sessions specifically eliciting his core values. It quickly became apparent that although he had clear values involving challenge, stimulation and creativity, he also had a strong set of values related to honesty, simplicity and spirituality – values not always found in abundance in the business world.

Once his core values became clear, it was easy to see why, although he was successful, he was deeply unsatisfied. We discussed ways in which he could meet the values that were not currently being met at work or in his spare time. He also recognised that while being involved in a company start-up met his values for challenge, stimulation and creativity, managing a business on a long-term basis left him with a sense of frustration and disappointment.

Finally, and most importantly, by understanding what mattered most to him in life, Alex had a clearer idea of what he was looking for in both his friendships and romantic relationships. The choices he has made since he developed this understanding mean that not only is he more fulfilled, he has begun to attract the right people into his life. Alex no longer feels lonely, even when he is on his own.

DISCOVERING YOUR CORE VALUES

From a very young age we are told what is right and what is wrong, what is good and what is bad, what matters and what doesn't. We are influenced by our parents and grandparents, our schools and community, and our religious and cultural background. As adults, we need to wade through these myriad influences and find out what really matters to us as individuals.

Covered later in this chapter is how to integrate your values with those of a partner, husband or wife, but first let's focus on working out what matters most to *you*.

As you begin to clarify your values, remember that one value is no more 'valuable' than another. It is important to know what your values are, to ensure that the choices you make in life are in alignment with them.

Be completely honest with yourself. If material possessions are truly important to you, be honest about it. Likewise, if it *really* matters that you get that corner office and Mercedes Benz, and your values include the importance of prestige, accept it. Not everyone can be satisfied with the life of a monk!

Your values are not an indicator of who you'd like to become or who you think you should be. They are simply a reflection of what matters to you – the person you are right now.

At different stages in life the expression of your core values may change. What mattered most when you were young, free and single may not be the key to your fulfilment when you are married with three children. At the same time, some values will never change. They are so deeply ingrained into who you are that all that changes as you progress through life is the choices you make to align yourself with these values.

Exercise

Work your way through the following list of life values.[*] Circle those you feel you strongly identify with.

ADVENTURE

Risk	The unknown	Thrill	Venture
Danger	Speculation	Dare	Exhilaration
Gamble	Endeavour	Quest	Experiment

BEAUTY

Grace	Refinement	Elegance	Taste
Attractiveness	Loveliness	Radiance	Gloriousness
Magnificence			

TO CATALYSE

Impact	Move forward	Touch	Alter
Turn on	Unstick others	Coach	Energise
Spark	Encourage	Influence	Stimulate

TO CONTRIBUTE

Serve	Improve	Augment	Provide
Assist	Endow	Strengthen	Foster
Facilitate	Minister to	Grant	Assist

TO CREATE

Design	Invent	Synthesise	Inspire
Imagination	Ingenuity	Originality	Assemble
Conceive	Plan	Build	Perfect

TO DISCOVER

Learn	Detect	Perceive	Distinguish
Locate	Realise	Uncover	Observe
Discern			

TO FEEL

Make	To experience	Sense	Sensations
To glow	To feel good	Be with	In touch with
Energy flow			

[*] Published with the permission of CoachU www.coachu.com

TO LEAD

Guide
Cause
Reign

Inspire
Arouse
Govern

Influence
Enrol
Rule

Model
Encourage
Persuade

MASTERY

Expert
Dominate field
Pre-eminence

Superiority
Greatest
Set standards

Primacy
Best
Excellence

Outdo
Adept
Supreme

PLEASURE

Have fun
Sensual
Be entertained

Be hedonistic
Bliss

Sex
Be amused

Sports
Play games

TO RELATE

Be connected
To unite
Be bonded

Part of the
community
To nurture

Family
Be linked with

Be with
Be integrated

BE SENSITIVE

Tenderness
Be present
Show compassion

Touch
Empathise

Perceive
Support

See
Respond

BE SPIRITUAL

Be aware
Relate with God
Honouring

Be accepting
Devoting

Be awake
Holy

Religious
Passionate

TO TEACH

Educate
Inform
Prime

Instruct
Prepare

Enlighten
Edify

Explain
Uplift

TO WIN

Prevail
Score
Triumph

Accomplish
Acquire

Attain
Win over

Attract
Predominate

Compile the words you have circled into a short list. The idea is to create a final list of 6–10 core values. Be vigorous with your selection. For example, if you have circled two items in the adventure category, make an effort to choose the one item that resonates most closely with you.

Once you have your final list, go through each value and describe what it means to you and why it is important that this value is met in your life. See if you can capture this as a single sentence. Remember, the same words will mean different things to different people, so it is important that you are clear about what each word really means to *you*.

Another method for uncovering your core values is verbal elicitation. This can be done with a partner or friend – someone you can be completely honest with. One of you can take the role of the coach, while the other person works to define their core values.

The 'coach' is to repeat the question 'What matters most to you in life?' Each time the question is asked, the 'client' writes the first word that comes into his or her mind.

Answer this question 10–15 times. You will know you have drawn out the majority of your core values when you become stuck for an answer about what *really* matters, or your answers start to become variations on the same value.

Create a shortlist of 6–10 items and go through this list describing what each value means to you, and why it matters in your life.

A PRESCRIPTION FOR LIFELONG FULFILMENT

Knowledge is power – the importance of understanding what your values are should never be underestimated. To really gain from this knowledge, however, you need to begin to live your life in a way that is directly aligned with your core values.

If your values are not being met you may feel you are not living up to your potential. You could find yourself successful but not satisfied, rich but lonely, or busy yet unfulfilled.

With your new understanding of what matters most, think about the life you are currently living. Are you truly fulfilled? Are some of your values being met? Do you feel that your life needs some slight tweaks, or is a complete overhaul required?

Now think about your dream life. Does the life you began to design through the exercises in Chapter 1 take you closer to or further from a life in which all of your values are being fully met? Would achieving this dream life leave you truly satisfied?

Understanding what really matters in your life, knowing your core values, and living your life in a way that is aligned to those values is a simple prescription for lifelong fulfilment.

Because your core values are likely to evolve through the different stages of your life, it's worthwhile completing the values elicitation exercise regularly. You might want to review your values each year, as part of your annual goal-setting process (see Chapter 5) or, at the very least, when your life is changing in a significant or fundamental way, such as leaving school or university, getting married, starting a family or when your children leave home.

Reviewing your core values as the years progress is also an interesting way to keep track of how your life is changing, and can provide an insight into the person you once were.

Understanding what really matters in your life is a simple prescription for lifelong fulfilment.

DECISION-MAKING MADE EASY

We all know how hard making life's most important decisions can be, but when we know our core values, decision-making suddenly becomes much easier.

Usually when we need to make a decision, we compare one alternative to another. We diligently write out our lists of 'for' and 'against', then wonder why we are no closer to understanding what the *right* answer is.

Trying to make decisions this way is like comparing apples and oranges while asking the question 'Which is the better fruit?' How much easier would it be if you took the time to understand what you needed from this fruit in order to be satisfied? You could then ask a different question altogether, such as which fruit is better for thirst quenching, making juice, baking or palate cleansing. The answers become obvious.

If you take a values-based approach to decision-making you have something to measure each alternative against. Your values are an indicator of what really matters in your life. By evaluating each option against your core values rather than against each other, you have a much clearer indicator of which one will leave you with a greater sense of fulfilment and satisfaction.

Having a clear understanding of your values means that you can start to look at your life as a whole. You will quickly be able to understand the benefits of one decision compared with another, and how each choice will affect your overall goal of creating your dream life.

Exercise

Go back to the list of core values you defined in the previous exercise. Next to each value, give yourself a score out of 10 – indicating how prevalent that value is in your life today. A score of 10 means that the value is being met in your life and there is nothing you could do to achieve a greater sense of satisfaction in this area. A score of 0 would mean, unfortunately, that the value is nowhere to be found in your life.

Look over your scores. For each value that currently scores below 7 out of 10, identify three things you could do, choices you could make or plans you could put into action to bring you closer to a life that is in alignment with your values.

WORK IS WHAT YOU DO, NOT WHO YOU ARE

In Western society today most adults spend at least 50 per cent of their waking hours working. Being clear about how we feel about our work, and understanding what does and does not matter to us when we are working, is vital if we are to find our work satisfying and fulfilling.

There are many different types of work, and when it comes to values we are not limited to the concept of paid work – it includes voluntary work, home-making, parenting and caring.

It is important to remember that work is one of the many things that we do with our time. It is what we do, not who we are. This means our work values are a subset of our overall life values, in the same way that we have family values, relationship values, financial values, and health and wellbeing values.

Because most of us do spend so much of our time engaged in the activity of work, understanding our values and working towards an *occupation* that is aligned with those values can not only increase our sense of satisfaction and fulfilment at work, it can also significantly increase our overall fulfilment and life satisfaction.

Understanding your work values can influence the choices you make and the way you go about it. Even when your work is unpaid, your values need to be considered if you want to make the most of this time and ensure that it is as fulfilling and meaningful as possible.

Most people find that their work values shift over time. When you are young, free and single it might be important that your work is flexible and provides plenty of time off for travel. As you take on more responsibilities, such as a car, mortgage or a family, the values relating to job security are likely to take on far greater importance.

It is important to evaluate your work values at regular stages, as well as assessing how the work you are currently doing measures up against your values. Something that appeared perfectly in alignment with your values at the interview stage may prove to be lacking a few years down the track.

Louise's story

Throughout her twenties Louise had been heavily focused on her career. On the fast track to becoming a partner at a top accounting firm, she knew that her career values revolved around achievement, prestige, reward and challenge. She knew what she wanted and she was willing to work for it. But what of her life values? For a long time Louise's life had been her work; she had believed that they were one and the same.

In her early thirties she married and gave birth to her first child. She had decided to take the minimum maternity leave and get back to work as soon as possible. She employed a full-time nanny and felt confident that her child was receiving the best possible care.

Although Louise had cut back on her working hours, her job was still demanding and regularly required her to take work home. When she first returned to work she felt she had it all sorted out, but later she stopped feeling so confident. She couldn't get over the nagging feeling that she was missing out on something.

When she talked to friends and family she got conflicting advice. Some said she should leave work to be a full-time mum and that this was the only path to fulfilment. Others said it was

(continued)

just her hormones and that she would get used to the corporate grind in no time at all. Others tried to be helpful and suggested all sorts of compromises. It seemed to Louise that whatever decision she made, she would be missing out on either motherhood or her career aspirations.

When she came to see me it was clear that Louise needed to spend some time working out her life values and realise that her job wasn't her *life* but rather something that she did with her life.

Louise hadn't questioned her work values in nearly 15 years. When she left university she had known what she wanted and had been so busy working towards it that she hadn't stopped to check if what she was working towards still had a high priority in her life.

Louise discovered that she had strong core values relating to family, togetherness and quality time, and that a significant factor in her frustration was that these values were in conflict with her work choices. She also found that while her work values still favoured success and achievement, they were now just an element of the bigger picture, not the whole picture.

Armed with this new self-knowledge, Louise was able to make decisions confidently about her work/family balance that would bring her a significant step closer to her overall satisfaction and fulfilment.

She has decided to work part-time for the next few years, and while she hasn't given up her plans for a partnership, she is happy to put them on the backburner until her son has started school.

Exercise

Read through the following list* of work values and rate each one with a score from 1 to 5:

1 This is always important to me.
2 This is often important to me.
3 This is sometimes important to me.
4 This is occasionally important to me.
5 This is never important to me.

Independence	Job tranquillity	Change and variety
Challenging problems	Creative expression	Fast pace
Exercise competence	Work under pressure	Aesthetics
Physical challenge	Status	Work on the frontier
Security	Precision work	Friendships
Intellectual status	Public contact	Influence people
Knowledge	Make decisions	Affiliation
Advancement	Help others	Power and authority
Excitement	Competition	Stability
Work alone	Help society	Creativity (general)

* Published with the permission of Career Trainer www.careertrainer.org

Community	Location	Family
Profit/gain	Time freedom	Fun and humour
Artistic creativity	Supervision	Work/life balance
Recognition	Work with others	Tradition
Adventure	Moral fulfilment	Steep learning curve
High earnings anticipated	Honesty and integrity	Personal safety
Spirituality	Diversity	Structure and predictability
Group and team	Practicality	Environment

If you find you have rated more than five or six items as category 1, feel free to create a sub-category: '1.5 – This is nearly always important to me.' It doesn't matter how many items are in each of the other categories – what you are focusing on is identifying your core work values.

While it may be unlikely that you will spend every waking hour of every working day being 100 per cent fulfilled, knowing your work values will mean that you spend a far greater percentage of each day satisfied with how you are spending your time.

DOING WHAT YOU'RE GOOD AT AND DOING WHAT YOU LOVE

Successful but still not satisfied? You could be doing work that you are good at, but don't particularly enjoy.

For most of us, our first career plans were made in high school, usually under heavy influence from our parents, teachers and friends. You're good at maths, why don't you become an accountant; good at English, become a journalist; talk a lot, become a barrister! These decisions are often made long before we have a chance to discover what we actually enjoy doing.

Many people dream of a perfect world in which they imagine themselves doing something they have little or no experience in, but which they truly believe they could be brilliant at if only they were given the chance. Just because you are good at something, it doesn't mean that engaging in that activity will be aligned with your values. You might be excellent at filing and administration, but this might not meet your values of creative expression and continual change. Likewise, you might be a deeply creative and talented musician, but working in a band may not meet your values of security and regular income.

There is another reason why doing what you are good at isn't always satisfying – sometimes it comes too easily to you. Many people find that being regularly challenged is an important source of stimulation and satisfaction, and doing what you know you can do in your sleep is not very challenging at all!

Exercise

First make a list of 10 things you do well. This might include things you know you are good at and things other people tell you you're good at.

Rate each activity on a scale of 0–10 where 10 is 'I am truly passionate about this activity' and 0 is 'I couldn't care less if I never did this again as long as I live!' Then look at all the items you scored 7 or above. How many of these do you currently spend your time doing? What simple changes could you make so you spend more time doing these things?

Now make a list of 10 things you love doing. This list can include things you are good at but never get a chance to do; things you are average at but wish you did better; and things you love doing but don't get the chance to do often enough to know if you are any good or not.

Again, rate each item on a scale of 0–10. This time 10 means 'I spend nearly all my time doing this' and 0 means 'I know I'd love doing this if only I got the chance!'

This time, look at all the items that score seven or below. What changes could you make in your work and your life so you spend more time doing the things that you love?

Finally, focus on the items you love doing but aren't particularly good at yet. Make a plan to improve, whether that means regular practice, additional training or studies, or simply making changes in your life that mean you get the chance to do these things more often.

THE QUEST FOR WORK/LIFE BALANCE

Work/life balance is the hot topic of our times. As companies demand more of their employees, and people begin to expect more luxuries in their lives, the hours we work become longer and longer.

Your core values can help you create and maintain a sense of balance in your life. When you know what matters most to you, you are much clearer about what you are actually working for.

If your work is consistent with your values, it stops feeling so much like work and the quest for work/life balance begins to become less important. You've probably heard the expression 'Do the work you love and you'll never work a day of your life'. Well, it's true. If you are engaged in activities you find stimulating and fulfilling, they cease to feel like work and start to feel like play!

Now this doesn't mean you should give up your desire for a balanced life and focus all your attention on doing one thing – that would hardly be healthy. After all, even if you love broccoli, you still need to eat a variety of vegetables if you are to maintain a healthy body. The same goes for your mind. But doing work you love does mean that you can stop splitting your life into work and other time, and start thinking of your occupation as just one of the many stimulating and satisfying things you engage in.

In a perfect world, work/life balance would not be an issue at all. We would simply spend all of our time doing things we love doing. The only difference would be that some of those activities generate an income and others expend that income.

RELATIONSHIP MATTERS

If you are married, in a partnership or have children, you might want to spend some time defining values for you as a couple or family. All successful relationships are based on compromise, and while this doesn't mean that you need to compromise your own personal values, it might mean that the values you agree on for your relationship are a compromise based on both your and your partner's personal values.

When you start a new relationship, having a solid understanding of your life and personal relationship values will give you a clearer picture of whether or not the new relationship has potential. If your values are in direct conflict with those of your partner, then it is unlikely that this will be a long and happy union. However, if your values are compatible – and they don't have to be identical, just compatible – you will have a much better chance of creating a lasting and successful relationship.

We have already explored how values continue to evolve and how they are directly influenced by each key life stage. This is particularly apparent when you have children.

In many cases, starting a family may require a complete renegotiation of what does and doesn't matter in your life. You and your partner need to work together on defining your family values. While it is important that you understand your own personal needs, if you are working towards creating a happy union it is important that you don't work in isolation. Instead, look at how you would like your family life to develop in a way that meets both partners' individual values, your values as a couple and your values as a family.

THE KEY TO *REAL* SUCCESS AND HAPPINESS

Having an understanding of your values is like having the key that unlocks the secret to a fulfilling life. If you know what makes you happy, what fulfils and satisfies you, and, just as importantly, what leaves you frustrated and dissatisfied, you can immediately begin to make changes in your life that will take you closer to your dream life.

By making the commitment to living a life that is in alignment with your values, you will have taken a big step towards making your dream life a reality.

If you live your life in alignment with your values, you have already begun to live your best life.

KEY LESSONS – UNDERSTANDING WHAT MATTERS

1. Your values are the DNA of your soul – they are the things that matter most to you in the world. Understanding your life values is the key to creating the life of your dreams.

2. No one value is more 'valuable' than another. Values are simply an honest expression of the things that are of most *value* to you.

3. When you understand your life values, decision-making will become much easier.

4. Work is what you do, not who you are. You need to consider your work values as a subset of your overall life values.

5. Make sure you do what you love. Just doing what you are good at won't guarantee your fulfilment.

6. To live a balanced life, make sure that you work towards meeting all of your values, not just one or two.

7. Relationship values and family values should be developed together with your partner. The values you agree on should be a compromise based on each of your personal values.

8. If you live your life in alignment with your values, you have already begun to live your best life.

CHAPTER 3
Eliminating limiting beliefs and behaviours

Are you living your best life? Are you realising your true potential? If not, why isn't your current life measuring up to your dream life?

Instead of looking around and coming up with a list of reasons why, start to look within and understand the role you play in holding yourself back from achieving everything that you want in your life.

I'm not saying there aren't some things in life that are well and truly beyond your control, but there is probably a lot more within your control than you realise. Simply by choosing to think different thoughts and develop new habits, you will find that achieving your true potential actually becomes easy.

ARE YOU HOLDING YOURSELF BACK?

'How do I hold myself back?' is one of the most powerful questions you can ask yourself. Do you know all the different ways in which you prevent yourself from achieving your true potential? When you were asked to suspend reality in Chapter 1 and think about a perfect world, did you find yourself saying, 'But that's not possible, that could never happen to me...'?

The way some people hold themselves back will be as simple as not truly believing they can achieve their goal. For others, a far more complex set of thoughts and actions is getting in their way.

If you want to create your dream life, then eliminating your limiting beliefs and behaviours must become a priority. You want nothing to hold you back as you work towards living your goal.

> **'How do I hold myself back?'
> is one of the most powerful questions
> you can ask yourself.**

A limiting belief is a thought that holds you back, a belief about yourself and your life that limits your potential. Limiting beliefs are sinister because although they are entirely subjective, our subconscious accepts them as fact, without questioning their validity.

Have you ever found yourself at a job interview thinking that you'll never get the job; or perhaps telling yourself you are fat and no one will ever find you attractive? Each time you have negative thoughts like these, you are sending your subconscious a very clear message that you are not worth success, love and happiness.

Exercise

Ask yourself the question: 'How do I hold myself back?' Make a list of all the things you say, think or do that get in the way of achieving your goals. Include everything you can think of, no matter how big or small. You might find it easier to break this question down into the key areas of your life: health and fitness; financial security; career; relationships; work/life balance; and home life.

If you think you have completed your list, ask yourself the question again – 'How do I hold myself back?' – and see what other answers come to you. You might need to go through this process two or three times before your list is complete.

Then make a note next to each item describing a simple change you could make to stop holding yourself back in this way. You'll come up with more ideas as you work through this chapter, but make a start on this exercise right away.

It can be quite a shock to discover all the different ways in which you have been compromising your own success, but don't let this list dismay you. Instead, look at it as a starting point: by uncovering all the ways you currently hold yourself back, you are so much closer to having the power to create your dream life!

When you set your sights on a goal, do you do everything in your power to make it possible? Do you do most things, some things, or even just a few things to bring your goal one step closer? Or do you let yourself slip up time and time again, continually making excuses for never achieving what you set out to do?

Every day you make different choices and these decisions have a direct impact on what you achieve in your life. It might be that you eat a big piece of cake, even though you have decided that you want to lose weight. Or perhaps you decide that it is too cold outside to exercise, when deep down you know that as soon as you get started you will begin to warm up.

If you have ever had similar thoughts, then you will need to work on eliminating your limiting behaviours. Discovering how you hold yourself back and putting in place strategies to eradicate each of your limiting beliefs and behaviours is a powerful step towards creating your dream life.

DEVELOP A POSITIVE PERSPECTIVE

The fastest way to your dream life is to develop a positive perspective – a view of the world that considers everything in the best possible light. Once you develop a positive perspective, you will quickly learn not to be concerned by little things. You will no longer worry about the ups and downs of everyday life. If you fundamentally believe that your life is a good one, every single day, regardless of what takes place, will simply be another wonderful day.

> **The fastest way to your dream life is to develop a positive perspective.**

Looking for the positive in every situation means that you no longer think of outcomes as good or bad. Instead, things have either gone your way the first time, or you have had the chance to learn something new, something that will make things easier the next time. And we all know that learning is a positive thing! When things feel hard, or are not going as easily as they should, apply your positive perspective and look for the learning opportunity

Another benefit of a positive perspective is that you become luckier. By seeing the positive or plus side of every situation, you are more likely to have an open mind and actually be in a position to seize opportunities as they present themselves. As the expression goes, 'The harder you work, the luckier you get'; well, the harder you work at being positive, the more you will be able to seize those 'lucky' opportunities as they appear.

Having a positive perspective doesn't mean that you ignore the cold, hard facts, nor does it mean you are ignorant of what some may see as the 'full picture'. A positive perspective is simply the angle of the picture you choose to focus on.

Being continually positive may take a bit of effort at first, especially if you are a cup half-empty type of person, but if you keep going you will find it will start coming naturally to you. On the rare occasions you do find yourself thinking negative thoughts, you will be able to replace them with more positive ones at the speed of light.

BE YOUR OWN CHEERLEADER

If you want to eavesdrop on an interesting conversation, start listening in to your inner dialogue, your self-talk. Everyone has a little voice in their head that is chattering away constantly. What kind of conversation is yours having?

You might find that your little voice is actually a big bully, constantly putting you down, criticising your efforts and telling you that you're just not good enough.

The conversations you have with yourself are some of the most important you will ever have. They are the basis for the continuing development of your self-esteem and confidence. After all, if you don't believe in yourself, how can you expect anyone else to?

The conversations you have with yourself are some of the most important you will ever have.

While it's important to be continually challenged and to strive to improve your performance, you might have fallen into the destructive habit of being your own worst critic. Listen in on the conversations you have with yourself. Are you generous, encouraging, inspiring and motivating; or are you critical, judgmental and downright mean? A good way of assessing your self-talk is to ask yourself whether you would ever speak that way to a friend. I doubt it – most people would be too considerate of their friend's feelings to be that cruel!

A good guide for self-talk is never to speak more harshly to yourself than you would to your own small child. It's quite an interesting thought. After all, a parent is the guardian of a child's self-esteem. As an adult, you are the guardian of your own.

When we engage in negative self-talk, not only do we erode our self-esteem and confidence, our subconscious actually believes everything we say

– as fact! Just think, every time you say to yourself 'Don't be so stupid', your subconscious believes that you *are* stupid.

One of the best ways to turn off your chattering voice – negative or simply noisy – is through meditation. Another is strenuous exercise. But what can you do when you are not huffing and puffing or chanting *om*? It is very difficult to get rid of your little voice altogether, but what you *can* do is decide once and for all who is boss and what conversations you are and are not willing to accept.

Exercise

Carry your journal with you for two to three days and make a note of your inner dialogue – the conversations you have with yourself. Write down the subject matter and nature of each conversation. Where negative conversations are concerned, stick to the subject of the conversation – I am not asking you to write down the negative beliefs. *Never* write down a negative belief. Confirming it in ink will only add to the power it already has to hold you back.

As you observe your inner dialogue you will start to see a pattern emerging. On some subjects you may find that you are your own harshest critic, and on others, hopefully, you will be your own cheerleader.

When you find yourself engaged in a negative internal conversation, stop it immediately. Take a moment to inject some positivity into your dialogue and practise being a cheerleader. If you keep this up, being your own cheerleader will starting coming naturally to you.

Make the decision to become your own cheerleader. Champion your good efforts at every turn, and on those odd occasions when you haven't been the best you can be, your inner cheerleader can focus on the valuable lessons you have learnt and how much better you are going to be next time.

LEARN TO REFRAME YOUR THOUGHTS

One of the easiest ways to eliminate your limiting beliefs is to reframe your thoughts. Reframing is a simple technique: take an existing negative or limiting thought, evaluate it objectively, then replace it with a more accurate, positive thought. This is a conscious process and one you can adopt at any time you find yourself expressing a negative statement about yourself, either verbally or within your internal dialogue.

Are you a harsh critic of your skills, abilities and potential? You probably learned this behaviour from the adults in your life while you were growing up. Perhaps your parents or teachers always criticised you, believing, incorrectly, that this was the best way to encourage you to give your best.

They were wrong. Don't let yourself be fooled into believing that harsh criticism ever gets the best results. To encourage someone, even yourself, to achieve excellence, provide positive, motivating and encouraging messages. Positive reinforcement always brings out the best in people.

If you find yourself engaging in a limiting thought, you need to replace it with a positive one – quickly! One of the easiest ways to do this is to ask yourself what an objective outsider or third party would think. What would someone who doesn't know you say about your performance or effort? Would they say that it wasn't very good, or would they see that you had put in a lot of effort, and that while there may be some room for improvement, you've made excellent progress?

The thought you would then use to replace your excessively critical thought would be 'I have put in a good effort and I have really improved', not 'I was nowhere near as good as I need to be'.

It's important that you get into the habit of replacing a negative thought with a positive or, at the very least, objective statement immediately – as soon as it comes into your head. The longer you let negative thoughts linger, the more damage they are doing to your self-esteem, confidence and, ultimately, your belief in your ability to achieve your goals.

This might be hard to do at first, but if you commit to reframing your negative thoughts quickly, you will soon find that reframing comes naturally to you. In fact, after a while you will have eliminated your negative thoughts altogether.

Ben's story

Ben was a division manager in a large manufacturing company. While he was growing up, his father had been strict about his schoolwork, telling him that he only wanted what was best for his son. Ben's father always told him that nothing but 100 per cent was acceptable. Anything less was simply not good enough. Even when Ben came home from school with a grade of 90 per cent, his father wanted to know where the other 10 per cent had gone!

At the same time, his father wanted to make sure he didn't become complacent or 'too big for his boots', so he was never permitted to acknowledge his success or be proud of his hard

(continued)

work. Ben's father wasn't a bad person; he was probably treating his son the same way his father had treated him and the only way he knew how.

While outwardly confident, Ben's early experiences had had a lingering and destructive effect on his self-esteem. He found himself constantly criticising his own work. Regardless of what his managers said, he didn't believe that anything he did was ever good enough. Even when he was given a promotion or pay rise he found himself wondering if he really deserved it.

Ben's manager asked him to think about seeing a personal coach. He explained that the company was very happy with his performance, and that the only thing holding him back in his career was his lack of belief in himself.

Ben and I began to work on building his self-esteem and confidence. He learned to reframe his limiting beliefs by looking at his performance through the objective eyes of an outsider. When challenged, Ben had to admit that he must be pretty good. He had been regularly promoted, always received top marks in his performance reviews and his managers frequently commended him on his efforts.

Slowly Ben learned to replace his negative thoughts with these new positive ones based on the simple, logical facts he was encouraged to observe. Over time his confidence and self-esteem grew. He continued to put in 110 per cent effort to everything he did, just like he always had, but now that he believed in himself, there really was nothing that could hold him back.

Exercise

Using logic and objectivity, begin to reframe any negative thoughts you identified in the previous exercise (page 63).

For each negative thought, try asking yourself the following questions:

- What would someone else say about this?
- What is the likelihood this is true?
- What would I say to someone who said this about himself or herself?
- Are there any examples where this might not be the case?

Now aim to diminish each negative thought by replacing it with a more accurate, positive thought.

REFORM YOUR THINKING WITH POWERFUL AFFIRMATIONS

The most powerful tool you can use to eliminate your limiting beliefs is to create an affirmation. Affirmations are simple, positive statements that reform negative thoughts by *affirming* as fact that which you wish to be true. Don't allow your negative thoughts to roam free in your mind. By repeating a set of positive statements or affirmations you will develop confidence in abundance.

Your subconscious is not 'intelligent'. It does not evaluate the messages it receives; it simply accepts them as fact. Your subconscious treats negative and positive messages equally. It influences your choices and actions, and does everything in its power to turn those messages into reality.

By repeating a set of positive statements or affirmations you will develop confidence in abundance.

There is nothing complicated about affirmations. They are simple, one- or two-line statements designed to fill your subconscious with positive messages so it can work towards making them a reality.

There are three simple rules for creating powerful affirmations:

1. *Positive.* There are no ifs, buts or maybes about affirmations. Likewise, there is no 'could', 'should' or 'I'll try'. For an affirmation to work it needs to be strong, powerful and *positive*.
2. *Present tense.* You want your subconscious to accept your affirmations as fact, so structure them in the present tense as if you have already achieved your goal. Use expressions like 'I have', 'I do' and 'I am'.
3. *Personal.* Your affirmations are powerless if they don't mean anything. When writing your affirmations, use words that excite and inspire you.

Write your affirmations down, then read or say them aloud as often as possible – every morning, every night and every spare moment in between! My minimum recommendation for affirmations is the 'rule of threes'. Say each affirmation three times at least three times per day. As I say, this is the minimum. The more you repeat your affirmations, the more powerful they become.

To make it easy to remember to say or read your affirmations you might like to use affirmation cards. I write down my affirmations on a card and leave it on my bedside table. I read it every morning and night. I have an affirmations card in between my PC and my telephone, so whether I am writing or talking I am always reminded of them. I also have an affirmations card in my wallet. Every time I spend money I am again reminded to say my affirmations.

There are lots of different things you can try to keep your affirmations at the front of your mind. Here are some of the techniques my clients use:

- Use your affirmations as the screensaver on your computer.
- Make your affirmations the screen saver on your personal organiser or mobile phone.
- Laminate your affirmations and stick them up on your shower wall.
- Stick them on your bedroom mirror.
- Use them as a bookmark in the book you are reading.

Whatever method you choose, what matters most is that you absorb these strong, positive messages on a regular basis. You will soon find they become a part of who you are.

Andrea's story

When Andrea's last relationship ended she was heartbroken. She had really hoped Dan would turn out to be 'the one'. They had been living together for nearly a year, but, unfortunately, what started out well quickly turned into constant fights and arguments. It seemed that once they were living together, they simply couldn't agree on anything.

As much as she loved Dan, Andrea could see that the relationship wasn't working. Dan had come to the same conclusion, announcing that he wasn't happy and wanted to move out.

(continued)

Andrea knew Dan was right, but it didn't make it any easier. Not only did she feel all the usual heartache associated with a break-up, she also felt foolish and angry with herself for thinking that she and Dan had what it takes. She came to coaching because she knew she was stuck in a rut of negativity and had started to feel sorry for herself. She had lost her confidence and didn't feel attractive anymore. She was worried she might never find the right man and that, although she was only 33, she would end up alone in her old age.

I asked Andrea to examine the limiting beliefs she had developed since the break-up, then explained how to create affirmations to support the progress she wanted to make in this area of her life.

Remembering that her affirmations needed to be positive, in the present tense and personal, Andrea chose the following:

- I am excited about my future.
- I recognise all my positive qualities and others recognise them too.
- I enjoy meeting new people and having the opportunity to get to know them.

Andrea got into the habit of saying each of these affirmations three times every morning and night as well as several times in between. Within weeks she felt like a new woman. Her sense of doom about her future had lifted and she had a spring in her step. She felt attractive again and it showed – she had been on several dates, one with a man who had 'potential'. Her confidence

(continued)

returned and she was no longer afraid of getting hurt in the future; she was having far too much fun in the present!

Exercise

Look back at the internal conversations you identified in the exercise on page 63. Where the dialogue was negative, see if you can work out the underlying limiting belief.

Next, I want you to work on designing an affirmation that both eliminates your limiting belief and supports you in living your best life. Make a note of this affirmation in your journal and commit to repeating it three times every morning, every night and at least one other occasion in between.

Repeat this exercise for at least three of your limiting beliefs.

Keep working with this same set of affirmations until you feel that they have taken effect and you have completely eliminated your negative belief.

UNCOVERING LIMITING BEHAVIOURS

Unlike our limiting beliefs, limiting behaviours actually result in an action, or lack of action, that has a direct impact on our progress. These behaviours hinder us and hold us back from achieving our potential.

While some limiting behaviours are deeply complex and could require help from a trained psychologist, most of the limiting behaviours I come across in my coaching practice are not complex and can be overcome simply by being aware that they exist. Here are some of my clients' most 'popular' limiting behaviours.

Limiting behaviour #1 – Believing that time will wait for you

You've heard the expression 'Time waits for no man' – well, it's true. It's important to realise that there will only ever be 60 seconds in every minute, 60 minutes in every hour and 24 hours in any one day. Unfortunately, it doesn't matter how much you try to squeeze into the available time, you will still be constrained by the amount of time that is available.

Many of my clients have claimed poor time management as the reason behind their lack of progress. The simplest thing you can do to improve your time management is to develop a healthy respect for time and the fact that it is never going to wait for you.

Limiting behaviour #2 – Thinking that worrying will make a difference

Worry is a particularly limiting behaviour – not only does it hold you back from action, it keeps you in a place of fear. There is absolutely nothing to be gained by worrying, ever! Things in life are either within your control – in which case you should do something about them – or beyond your control – in which case no matter how much worrying you do, it won't make a single bit of difference.

Limiting behaviour #3 – Waiting until you have enough money

I've heard from many people that they will do this or that – change careers, go back to studying, start a family – when they have enough money. But how much money is enough? While I am not encouraging financial recklessness, waiting until you have enough money is a losing game. You might find that the more you have, the more you spend, so you never end up feeling like you have enough.

If your goal really does require funding, get active and create a plan that will help you source or save the amount of money you need. Waiting won't achieve anything.

OVERCOMING LIMITING BEHAVIOURS

The most important step in overcoming your limiting behaviours is to own up to them. Take a good, honest look at yourself and the choices you make each and every day. Ask yourself if your actions really are the most effective way to achieve your goals.

It's not complicated. Once you have identified your limiting behaviours, create new habits or actions to replace them.

> **The most important step in overcoming your limiting behaviours is owning up to them.**

ARE YOU YOUR OWN WORST ENEMY?

Self-sabotage is a limiting behaviour in a different league altogether. When you self-sabotage you make choices – although they may not feel like choices at the time – that actively prevent you from achieving your goal. Some examples of self-sabotaging behaviour include getting drunk the night before a big job interview, being unfaithful when you are in a committed relationship, having a credit card blowout when your goal is to get out of debt, or binge eating when your aim is to lose weight.

On a subconscious level, self-sabotage is a way to prevent yourself from achieving your goals, by ensuring that your success is no longer possible or, at the very least, is now a long way off. The emotion behind every act of self-sabotage is fear – fear of success. Chapter 9 covers fears in detail, but for now it's important to know that when we self-sabotage, on some level we are afraid of the impact that achieving our goal will have on our lives. Subconsciously we do our best to prevent it from happening.

- Getting drunk before a big job interview might mean you are afraid of the increased responsibility and pressure to perform you will experience if you are given this new role.
- Being unfaithful may indicate a fear of not being good enough, or believing that you don't deserve to be this happy, so you engage in self-sabotage to hurt the relationship before it has the chance to hurt you.
- Blowing out on your credit card might indicate a fear of growing up, or of the new financial responsibilities you intend to take on when your debt is paid off, such as a mortgage.
- Bingeing when your weight loss is progressing well could be the result of a fear of being found attractive by the opposite sex, making you emotionally vulnerable and at risk of getting hurt.

If you find yourself engaged in self-sabotage, ask yourself, 'At what level is this behaviour working for me? At what level am I *supporting* a hidden fear of success?' If you can't discover this answer on your own, you might find it worthwhile to talk to a trained psychologist or counsellor.

IF YOU BELIEVE IT, YOU CAN ACHIEVE IT

The most important reason for identifying and eliminating your limiting beliefs and behaviours is that they have a direct impact on your ability to achieve your goals. The power of belief has been widely documented and you may have heard the expression 'Be careful what you wish for, it might come true'. The truth is, if you believe it, you can achieve it. This is precisely why it is so important that your beliefs are positive, motivating and designed to support you as you live your very *best life*.

KEY LESSONS – ELIMINATING NEGATIVE BELIEFS AND BEHAVIOURS

1. Don't blame the world for your lack of progress. Instead, look inside and ask 'How am I holding myself back?'
2. When you adopt a positive perspective you will no longer see things as good or bad; instead, you will see opportunities to learn a little or a lot!
3. Don't be a critic, be a cheerleader. Champion your efforts at every opportunity.
4. You are the guardian of your self-esteem. Never speak to yourself more harshly than you would to a small child.
5. If you find yourself being critical or demanding of your performance, examine your behaviour from an objective viewpoint. Imagine what an independent third party might say.
6. Positive, present tense and personal affirmations are *powerful* – use them!
7. Eliminating your limiting beliefs might be as simple as owning up to them. Overcoming self-sabotaging behaviours might need the help of a professional.
8. Spend time developing positive beliefs. If you believe it, you can achieve it!

CHAPTER 4
Creating a vision for your future

Are you ready to begin designing your future?

By now you have spent plenty of time dreaming about what your future could be like, and you are well and truly ready to start turning those dreams into reality.

The next step in creating the life of your dreams is to develop a *fine-tuned vision* of your future – a vision for the best life that you can possibly live.

Vision can mean many things. A glance at any dictionary will show that vision is, among other things: the ability to see; a vivid mental image produced by the imagination; and a great perception of future development.

By the end of this chapter you will have created a vivid mental image, one that will give you a sense of how your future is going to develop. The vision you create will provide you with purpose and direction — soon you really will be able to see where you are going.

Creating a vision for my own future was a major turning point in my life. From then on, I went from living a good, yet ordinary life to moving closer day by day to finding real success and happiness — to living my best life.

Having a vision gave me clarity and a sense of purpose that enabled me to live my life with ease, knowing that as long as I stayed true to my vision, each step I took would be taking me closer to the life of my dreams. By working towards my vision, I became one of those people for whom life appears simple. And it's true: life feels so much easier when you have a sense of purpose and direction, when you know what you are working towards.

I had an interesting conversation with a friend when I first started writing this book. I had just accepted an offer from my publisher and was excitedly telling my friend what the future held. This friend was in the process of downshifting. She had resigned from the paid workforce and was planning to spend her time at home, caring for her young son. It was something she had always wanted to do, but in the past her worries about money had prevented her from making this major life change.

After telling me how pleased she was for me, she said, 'You must really think I'm going nowhere...' I couldn't tell her fast enough how wrong she was! I was just as excited about her future as she had been about mine — after all, in working out that she didn't want the job she had, and actively working towards creating her best life, she was one step closer to living the life of her dreams. I quickly told her that I felt she was just as successful as I was — we just had different dreams.

DO YOU NEED A BLUEPRINT FOR YOUR FUTURE?

The short answer is no. You could happily exist for the rest of your life without ever taking the time to develop your vision. Would you be content in your life? Maybe. But do you really want to leave living your most meaningful and fulfilling life to chance? Would you run the risk of creating a life in which you simply 'exist'?

By creating a clear vision for your future you are taking ownership of your life. You are saying, 'This is what I want from life. This is what I need in my life if I am to achieve *real* success and happiness.'

If you haven't worked on your vision of the future before, it can be a little daunting at first. With pen in hand, you suddenly realise that the way you live your life is entirely up to you; that everything you have ever hoped and dreamed about could really be yours. What if you get it wrong? What if you fail? What if it's all a pipedream?

> **By creating a clear vision for your future you are taking ownership of your life.**

Although you will learn more as you read on about how to build your confidence and overcome your fears, for the time being I encourage you to take a leap of faith and trust that the future is yours for the taking.

When you create a vision, you are in effect designing a blueprint for your future. Your vision is the starting point from which your plans for future success and happiness can develop. With a clear vision in mind, you will be able to move calmly through each day, comfortable with the direction in which your life is going, and confident in the knowledge that you have created a foundation for your future.

Combined with the powerful discoveries you made when you explored your values, having a clear vision will render decision-making easier than ever. Not only will you know what matters to you, you will also know where you are heading. Every time you are presented with a set of options that require a decision, you will be able to ask yourself:

- Does this matter to me?
- Does this take me one step closer to my dreams?
- Which option will allow me to live in alignment with my values and move towards my vision for my future?

With this powerful knowledge, so many things in life will become much clearer and more simple.

If you have worked on creating a vision before, I advise you not to pick up an old vision and run with it. Instead, work through all the exercises in this chapter and make sure that the vision you are committing to is not just for any life, but for the life *you* have always dreamed of.

Exercise

Look back over your dream life and compile a shortlist of everything you would *really* like to have in your life. You have already eliminated all the things deep down you know are fantasies. Now I want you to make sure that even if you don't know how to go about getting these things in your life just yet, you are at least *willing* to work towards achieving them.

Once you have your list of all the key elements of your best life, I want you to review this list against your core values and ask yourself the following two questions: Is each item on your list in alignment with your core values. Are each of your values being met?

When you have finished this exercise, you should have a shortlist of all the elements that make up your vision.

THE IMPORTANCE OF KNOWING WHAT YOU DON'T WANT

Knowing what you *don't* want is just as important as knowing what you *do* want. Just like the 'old' life that I described in the introduction, lots of things can look good on paper. But until you have explored your dreams and identified your values, you have no real way of knowing if they are right for you. When you are living a life that isn't right, you are left with a constant sense of discomfort and frustration regardless of how successful you might appear. I used to describe it as feeling as if I was living someone else's life.

Having a clear vision will help you to ensure that you are *really* successful in all that you do. The success you experience will mean something to you, and you won't be left feeling successful but never satisfied.

If knowing what you don't want is to be a positive and useful piece of information, not just an opportunity to whinge or make knee-jerk changes in your life, then it's important to be very clear on why it is that you don't want it.

Understanding the real reason why something is not part of your vision can be invaluable, saving you from chasing unfulfilling fantasies and freeing up your time and energy to focus on what is really going to make you happy.

There is no place for 'could', 'should' or 'have to' in your vision. Make sure that the future you are creating doesn't include things you feel you ought to be doing to keep other people happy or to fulfil some outdated ideas of what your adult life should be like. This is your chance to start creating the life of your dreams, so make sure that you leave behind all the influences of your childhood, family or current work environment.

Knowing what you *don't* want is just as important as knowing what you *do* want.

The vision you are constructing needs to be one that will bring you real success and happiness — one that will serve as a blueprint for creating the life of your dreams.

Exercise

For the first part of this exercise, I want you to look back over the things you included in the first perfect-world exercise (page 25) and make a note of everything that didn't make it onto your vision elements list. Next to each item, I want you to acknowledge the reason why you know, deep down, that this does not belong in your vision. It might be that you wouldn't be willing to work for it, or that the compromises required would be too great, or that it would be in conflict with one of your core values.

Next I want you to make a list of 5–10 things that you have often felt you *should* want, have or do in your life, but that you know do not belong in your vision for your dream life. These might be things that other people have pressured you to consider, or that your culture, environment or family have influenced you into thinking are right for you.

Again, make a note next to each point describing why you know it is not the right thing for you.

For me, at the top of this list is 'become a lawyer'. My dad would have loved it if I had chosen this profession, but deep down I always knew it wasn't the right career for me. And while I would have enjoyed the performance element of being a barrister, I wasn't willing to commit to the years of study. I also believe that an environment focused on conflict, or even conflict resolution, would have exhausted my spirits.

Once you have completed this list, you can forget about all the things you don't want in your life – forever.

Andrew's story

In his late thirties, Andrew was the owner of a successful catering business. Although his business had always thrived, it had remained a small concern with six loyal staff. For various reasons, the previous year had seen business boom and several contracts were now coming Andrew's way – which would give him the chance to triple his profits.

At first Andrew was thrilled by this change and felt that he had finally 'cracked the big time', but for a few months he been feeling increasingly stressed. The constant worry in the pit of his stomach was starting to have a negative impact on his health and his personal life.

Andrew came to coaching because he wanted to explore why, when he had what he thought he had always wanted, he wasn't enjoying his work anymore.

Through coaching Andrew was able to see that it was largely external pressure that had led him to expanding his business, and that *his* vision for his future *did not* include him working long hours in a stressful environment. In Andrew's vision he had plenty of time for his family and he never took work worries home.

With coaching Andrew was able to see that although he was now more *financially* successful, he didn't feel successful because he was no longer able to meet his other life values.

With this discovery, Andrew developed a plan to scale his business back, confident in the knowledge that by focusing on what success meant to him, he would be able to enjoy his *whole* life a lot more.

CREATING YOUR VISION STATEMENT

Most companies have a vision statement – a couple of sentences expressing where the company is heading and what it intends to become. This vision statement is designed to be a compelling description of the future of the organisation that can be used both to create a sense of clarity about the company's purpose and to motivate and inspire its staff.

A personal vision statement works in much the same way, providing clarity as to your direction and what you want your life to be like. A personal vision statement will also help to motivate and encourage you as you work towards creating the life of your dreams.

When you have created your statement it will be as though you have created a master plan or road map for your future. You will still need to work out the details – when to turn left and when to turn right – but you will be clear on the overall direction you want your life to go in.

Lack of direction or purpose is one of the biggest causes of stress in modern life. So often when we are frustrated and dissatisfied, it is because we are drifting. It's not that we are going nowhere, but more that we are going nowhere particularly special!

When you have a clear vision, you will be able to set your sails and start heading in exactly the right direction for you.

A personal vision statement will help to motivate and encourage you as you work towards creating the life of your dreams.

Exercise

Go back to the list of key elements for your vision you identified earlier (page 27). It's likely that this shortlist falls generally into the categories of home life, relationships, work, money, health, recreation, and so on.

For each category, create a concise statement that captures the essential elements required to describe your vision. Here's an excerpt from my own vision statement:

My life is filled with people who I love and cherish. I have a dynamic social circle and I spend my time with people who are both stimulating and supportive.

Although a company's vision statement might be just two or three sentences, you might want to write a little more – after all, we are talking about your *entire* life here!

On the other hand, you might find that at the end of this exercise you want to write a simple sentence or two that summarises your whole life vision.

I have a single sentence that summarises my vision for all my professional pursuits:

I communicate the importance of creating the life you love to the widest possible audience.

Whether I am working on my next book or a magazine column, speaking at a conference or working one-to-one with a client, I constantly ensure that I am being true to my vision.

By creating your own vision statement, you will always know what you need in your life to experience *real* success and happiness.

You can look at creating your dream life in much the same way as you would look at building your dream home. You need to start by being clear on what you want – the number of bedrooms, the overall style of the architecture, whether it will be made of brick, stone or timber. Having a vision statement can be likened to briefing the architect designing your dream home. You might not know how many bricks you need, and you certainly don't have to know where you will be buying the bathroom taps, but you will have a clear idea of all the elements this house needs to have if it is to be the home of your dreams.

By taking the time to create your own vision statement, you will have a starting point, something to work towards, and a tool to help you recognise whether or not you are on track. You won't need to look outside to find sources of encouragement and motivation. You will know exactly what it is that motivates and inspires you, and you will be able to see how all of those elements tie together to create a life that is deeply satisfying and fulfilling.

LEARNING TO TRUST YOUR VISION

Whenever I do a visioning exercise I feel excited and inspired. In fact, I have learned the hard way not to do my visioning at night or I find I can't sleep – I'm much too excited by the future I am creating!

When you are writing your vision it's important to remember that it doesn't matter if you don't know how you are going to achieve it. The next chapter is dedicated to creating real and specific goals, which will form the building blocks of your vision.

You might already have some ideas about what you need to do, and if that's the case, brilliant! Write them down so you don't forget them. But, most importantly, don't get bogged down on the 'how' right now. All you need to do is have faith that the future you are designing really is a possibility. Make sure that you don't let any fears you may have about not knowing how to achieve your vision get in the way of your visioning exercises.

It requires courage to take control of your life, to decide not to accept just any future and instead create one that will fulfil your deepest desires. It is so much easier to be complacent; to go with the flow and just accept whatever life hands out. But if you really want to live the life of your dreams, you will need to be brave.

Very few of us can actually see into the future. So unless you are genuinely psychic, you will always be staring at the unknown when you consider your future. But if you work on creating your vision, you have less to be afraid of than if you drift along aimlessly. When you have a vision, you can be much clearer about the direction you want to go in, and you will be able to make conscious decisions that will lead you closer to a satisfying and fulfilling life.

I can't promise you that you will achieve every single element of your vision. I don't have a magic wand or a crystal ball, but I do know, with 100 per cent certainty, that if you take the time to form a clear vision and work towards bringing that vision into your reality, you will start to love your life.

BEING CONFIDENT ABOUT YOUR FUTURE

Some people find that creating a vision stirs up some uncomfortable feelings and worries that on some level they are not good enough and don't deserve the life described in their vision. If you are one of those people, I have a very simple message for you: *you deserve it!* You really do deserve to have the life of your dreams.

If you are feeling like this, the easiest way to overcome your doubts is to read your vision over and over again. If you read your vision statement again and again it will stop seeming like a fantasy and will start to feel like the most natural future you can imagine.

The idea is to create a sensation that your vision extends to a cellular level – your vision feels so natural to you, it's as if every cell in your body is working towards making it a reality.

Exercise

One of the most powerful techniques to support yourself in creating the life of your dreams is to focus on your vision – regularly and often. Try each of the following exercises to see which one works best for you – or combine all three – to make sure you have the best possible chance of making your vision a reality.

1. Read your vision statement aloud three times every morning when you wake up and every night before you go to sleep. You will find that before long you can almost recite it from memory. If you find yourself starting to feel complacent about your vision, mix up the order in which you read out your statements. Try starting from the end or the middle.

2. Print or write out several copies of your vision statement and stick them in places you know you'll see them on a regular basis. Every time you see your statement, read it through. Some places you might want to consider are:

- a bookmark in your diary
- on your bathroom mirror
- on your bedside table

   I have my vision statement stuck on the wall next to the door of my office. Every time I walk past, I read my vision and I am excited and inspired by what the future holds.

3. If you are losing confidence in your ability to achieve your vision, one of the best things to do is write it out, long hand, over and over, until it feels like there is simply no other alternative in your life.

Melanie's story

Melanie, a dynamic and motivated woman in her early thirties, was experiencing significant success at work, but deep down she knew that her current path wasn't fulfilling and was really only keeping her happy on the surface.

Initially, when Melanie and I began to discuss her vision for her future, she said she felt foolish and ungrateful for not being happy with what she had. I asked her to put aside these feelings for a while and just explore what her vision for the future might contain. She immediately identified that if she was living her dream life, not only would she be successful in whatever career she chose, but she would also be in a loving partnership and the mother of two children. As Melanie was single at the time, she laughed and said she felt that planning a future that included children when she didn't

(continued)

even have a partner was surely a waste of her time. I explained to her that the opposite was true and that it was important for her to visualise what her dream life would be like, regardless of whether or not she had the current resources to achieve it.

At first, when Melanie had completed her visioning exercises, which included a dynamic career as a writer and publisher and plans for romance and family, she said she actually felt down because it all seemed so far away.

I asked her to write down her vision and read it aloud three times every morning, every night and any time in between when she found herself doubting that her vision could be possible. I instructed her to do this for two weeks and report back at her next coaching session. Two weeks later I barely recognised the woman who walked through the door. She appeared taller and slimmer, younger yet wiser, and with a radiant smile.

Melanie had been diligently repeating her vision statement aloud and had found that, very quickly, the future she was designing for herself seemed like the most natural thing in the world. She even said that she could no longer remember all the fears and concerns she had felt when she first wrote down her statement.

By focusing on and affirming her vision, Melanie had developed a new-found confidence in her future. She now believed, deep down, that everything in her life was going to turn out exactly the way she wanted. She had complete confidence in her future and felt motivated and inspired to do whatever she needed to do to make this vision her reality.

VISUALISING YOUR VISION

A good way to support yourself in the achievement of your vision is to create vivid mental images or visualisations.

You may already have used visualisation techniques when you worked through the exercises in Chapter 1, but at that stage your visioning may have included your fantasies as well as the things you would genuinely like to see in your life.

Being able to create a visual blueprint for your future is just as important as creating a written or verbal one. Some people may be able to close their eyes and see the life of their dreams unfold before them. Others may need a little more help in seeing what their ideal future actually looks like.

Now that you know the elements contained in your vision, keep an eye out for images that support it. This might include pictures in magazines, advertising campaigns, artworks and postcards — any image that captures your attention and feels like a visual cue for the future you are working to create. Start a collection of these images; you might like to pin them to a board in your office or study, or if you are feeling creative you might like to build a vision map — a collage of all the images that support and inspire your vision.

I have one client who stuck all her vision images around her bedroom mirror, like a picture frame. Each day as she dresses and looks in the mirror, it is as if she is already living inside her vision.

You might want to create an 'inspiration and aspiration' folder to hold images and articles about things, people and places that excite and inspire you. In effect this becomes a resource book for your imagination, and as you are visualising your future you will have a rich library of images and ideas to draw on.

Exercise

Although you should visualise your dream life as often as possible in an informal way, there is a lot to be gained by making it a ritual. Sit in a comfortable and happy place. This might be your favourite armchair at home or under your favourite tree at a local park. Scent and sound are a great support to the imagination, so you might want to light a candle, burn some incense, listen to music or simply take deep breaths and inhale the air around you.

Once you have set up your environment, close your eyes and imagine you are living the life of your dreams. Imagine one day in this life in as much detail as possible. How do things look and feel? What are you wearing? What can you smell, what food can you taste, who do you spend your time with, and what feelings do you have as you go through your day?

You can completely lose yourself in this exercise, so make sure you do it when you are not going to be disturbed, and not when you are waiting for your bus or train to stop!

When you have exhausted every aspect of this exploration, open your eyes and write down in your journal as much as you can remember.

This is a wonderful exercise and you don't have to limit yourself to doing it just once! The more time you can spend visualising your ideal future, the more it will feel like a natural inclusion in your reality. Aim to find time to do this visualisation exercise for either five minutes each day or ten minutes two to three times a week.

Regularly visualise yourself within the life of your dreams. At first you might feel a little foolish, but soon you will be able to find a rich sanctuary in your mind – a place to go to remind you how wonderful your future is going to be.

SEEING INTO THE FUTURE

Although you might not be able to see literally into the future, by having a clear vision you can see the future you want to create for yourself. You will be able to see what every aspect of your life could potentially look like if you are willing to work for it.

Short of taking a psychic development course, the best way to see into your future is to start creating it. By having a clear sense of your vision, not only can you start making decisions that bring you closer to the future you are working to create, but you will feel confident in the knowledge that you are not just living any life, you are living your best life!

Each day we are faced with a continual stream of choices. Some are obviously significant – like an offer for a new job or the start of a new romance – but others are far more subtle: whether you walk to work or take the train; buy new shoes or save your money; the way you handle a difficult co-worker or an argument with a close friend or loved one.

Each of these scenarios presents you with a choice. Most of the time there isn't really a right or a wrong choice, but if you have a clear vision, you will know exactly what the right choice is for *you*.

With a clear vision you will never have to worry about making the right decision again – the answer will always be obvious. While you have no way of knowing exactly how things will turn out, you will be confident in the knowledge that you have made the choice that was most supportive of your future success and happiness.

> **With a clear vision you will never have to worry about making the right decision again – the answer will always be obvious.**

LIVE YOUR VISION TODAY

Knowing your vision for the future can also have a great impact on the way you live now. Take a moment to consider the way you currently live your life and the everyday decisions you make, and see what you can do to bring your vision for the future closer to the present.

In your vision, you might live in a home filled with fresh flowers. Bringing that future closer to your present might be as simple as spending the money you normally spend on a bottle of wine or a few drinks after work on a small bunch of flowers. Perhaps you have a personal trainer in your vision who meets you every morning to make sure you get the most out of your exercise regime. Consider sharing a trainer with two or three friends once a week. Again, in a simple and inexpensive way, you would be bringing your future closer to your present.

If your vision includes working flexible hours to spend as much time as possible with your children, bring a little of this future into your current reality by making simple changes such as starting work one hour later once a week so you can walk your children to school.

Many changes you can make to bring you closer to your vision won't cost you very much, but you might need to invest in a little extra planning and effort. Simple choices like these can have an amazing impact on your sense of fulfilment in your present life and can help encourage and motivate you to keep working towards creating the life of your dreams.

CLOSE YOUR EYES AND YOU WILL SEE!

Consider your vision as a way of seeing a life you don't yet have, but are completely committed to achieving in the very near future. At the visioning stage, it is not important to know how you are going to achieve your vision. All you need to know is that, at least as a concept, it is achievable.

You have already eliminated aspects that are just fantasies and what you really don't want or need to have in your dream life. Now it's time to concentrate your energies on what you believe is possible.

The next few chapters look at exactly what you need to do if you are to achieve your vision. The more you focus on your vision and visualise your future, the more real it will seem. If you are willing to combine that focus with effort and commitment, your vision will soon become your reality.

KEY LESSONS – CREATING A VISION FOR YOUR FUTURE

1. Take ownership of the direction of your life. Create a vision then work towards making it your reality.

2. If you want to create *real* success and happiness in your life it is important to know what you *don't* want in your life.

3. Lack of direction is one of the biggest causes of stress in life. When you create your vision, you capture exactly what motivates and inspires you and you know what you are working towards.

4. It requires courage to take control of your life and not just accept *any* future.

5. Repeat or affirm your vision until you believe it at a cellular level. You want to feel as though every cell in your body is working towards making your vision a reality.

6. Spend time visualising your future. Being able to create a visual blueprint for your future is just as important as having a written or verbal one.

7. If you know what your vision is, decision-making becomes easy. Evaluate each option on the basis of whether it takes you closer to or further from your dream life.

8. Look at your present life and see what simple, inexpensive changes you can make. Start living your dream today!

Step 2

KNOW **WHAT** YOU NEED TO DO

CHAPTER 5
Designing real and specific goals

Several research studies have shown that only one in ten people sets specific goals and that an even smaller percentage writes those goals down and commits to achieving them. In one particularly well-known study, conducted by Yale University in 1953, students were asked if they had written down their goals. Only 3 per cent answered yes. After twenty years, the participants were contacted again. The research found that the 3 per cent who had written down specific goals had amassed more material wealth that the remaining 97 per cent put together!

Of course money is not the only measure of success, but from a research point of view, it's useful because it is both tangible and objective.

It's fairly safe to assume that if there were a quantifiable, objective measure for happiness, satisfaction or fulfilment then the group that sets goals in these areas would more likely to achieve them.

OK! So the research suggests that goal-setting is generally a good idea, but why should you set goals? Having a goal can help you find your way – from where you are now to where you would like your life to be. Goals are like stepping stones from the present to the life of your dreams.

At its simplest, a goal is a positive statement about something you would like to do, be or have. But don't let the simplicity fool you. Goals are some of the most powerful tools to inspire, encourage and motivate you to achieve *real* success and happiness.

Some people find that when it comes to writing down their goals, they feel pressured or stressed – as if somehow they are setting themselves up to fail or feel disappointed. Writing down your goals is actually one of the most powerful things you can do, and the exercises in this chapter will show you how to set and write goals in a way that feels natural. You might even find the whole process exciting – I know I do!

Goals are some of the most powerful tools to inspire, encourage and motivate you to achieve *real* success and happiness.

QUICK WINS AND SHORT-TERM GOALS

All goals can generally be broken down into short-, medium- and long-term. Some of the goals you will set to help you work towards achieving your vision and creating *real* success and happiness are likely to be long-term. Other goals that involve changes that can be achieved sooner rather than later are likely to be short-term.

As a guide, your short-term goals are things that you will achieve in the next three months, medium-term goals will be achieved over the next twelve months, and long-term goals over the next three to five years. There is absolutely no prescription for this, and these terms are really just a guide to help create some structure around your goal-setting.

One of the most effective ways to create a dramatic improvement in your current life and move a big step closer to your best life is to set some simple short-term goals that you know you can quite easily achieve if you put your mind to it. In the business world these are called 'quick wins', and if you think about it, whatever your short-term goals are, achieving them will make you feel like a winner! A quick comparison of your current life with your dream life will tell you exactly what short-term goals and quick wins you can put into place.

If, on the other hand, your dream life is far removed from your current reality and you feel like you don't know where to begin, the Wheel of Life exercise will help you work this out (see page 106).

It really doesn't matter where you begin setting your goals or quick wins; what matters is that you do it! Once you get started and begin to enjoy the benefits of these simple but effective changes in your life, you will be inspired with more ideas for other short-term goals and quick wins.

Exercise

One of the easiest exercises to help you decide which areas of your life to focus on first is the Wheel of Life. This will give you a quick insight into the short-, medium- and long-term goals you need to set if you are to achieve *real* success and happiness.

Draw a circle and split it into eight segments. Label each segment with one of the following key life areas: friends; family; significant other or romance; health and fitness; work and career; fun and recreation; finance and money; and personal growth or spirituality. Using the centre of the wheel as 0 and the outer edge as 10, mark your level of satisfaction with each life area by drawing a line across that segment.

The Wheel of Life represents balance, and ideally you want your wheel to be pumped up to at least 8 out of 10. If your wheel is looking a bit like a flat tyre, you will know exactly where your goal-setting needs to begin. Ask yourself the following questions:

- What would I need to do/be/have or change if I was to move this segment from its current score to at least an 8 or 9 out of 10?
- What quick wins or short-term goals could I put in place that would move this segment at least one point closer to being a fully pumped tyre?

Use your answers to these questions to set at least three short-term goals, three medium-term goals and three long-term goals.

Even though the changes you are making in your day-to-day life might seem simple, the results can make a dramatic improvement in how you feel about your life as a whole.

HOW 'SMART' DO YOU NEED TO BE?

You might have heard about the simple formula for ensuring that your goals are intelligent and powerful, not just wishes on a breeze. For your goals to be most effective, you need to make them SMART goals:

Specific. Be as precise as you possibly can be with your goal-setting. Don't just say 'I want a new car', say 'I have a brand-new shiny black Mercedes Benz 500 SL'. Provide as much detail as you need to create the most vivid picture of what you want to bring into your life.

Measurable. How are you going to know when you have achieved your goal? It's really important to set measurable goals. While the example of a new car is already measurable in that the goal is to have a car, for other goals that don't have an inherent measurement you must quantify what it is you are setting out to achieve. If you want to lose weight, say how many kilograms or pounds you would like to lose. If you want to save money, create a specific target. If your goal is to increase the turnover of your business, list a percentage increase or a monetary figure.

Achievable. Is it actually possible to achieve your goal? If my goal were to be a prima ballerina, in my mid-thirties, with no ballet training, I think we would all agree that my goal might fail this test. Test that your goal is not a pipedream. In your heart you need to believe that, if you apply the right degree of effort and create a good plan, you can definitely achieve your goal.

Realistic. 'Realistic' and 'achievable' may seem one and the same, but there is a difference. 'Achievable' is used to mean whether or not something is generally possible; 'realistic' refers specifically to you and whether this goal can feasibly be achieved in your life. What compromises are you willing to make to achieve your goal and what constraints or restrictions do you currently face? While it might be perfectly achievable to run a marathon, it might not be realistic for you if you have recently had knee surgery. Likewise it could be perfectly achievable, based on your background, to become CEO of a major corporation, although not realistic if you plan to work only six months of the year.

Time-based. The 'when' question! It's important that as you set goals, you also determine the time frame in which you intend to achieve them. Your time scales may be influenced by your responses to both your assessment of what is achievable and what is realistic. It doesn't matter if you are unsure exactly how long it will take to achieve your goals – unless you have a crystal ball you probably can't be – but it's important that your estimation is as accurate as you can make it, given the available information.

THE RULES – POSITIVE, PRESENT TENSE AND PERSONAL

Having confirmed that your goals are SMART, there are only three simple rules you need to remember. Goals, just like affirmations, should be positive, present tense and personal.

Rule #1 Positive

Designing goals requires positivity. You need to express your goals in the most positive form possible. Don't say 'I hope', 'I'll try', 'I wish', or 'one day'. Say '*I have*', '*I am*' and '*I do*'.

Rule #2 Present tense

Designing your goals also requires using your imagination. Describe your goals as if they have already happened. If you want to change jobs, don't say 'Hopefully I will get a new job.' Say '*I have a new job*'. Likewise if your goal is to meet your life partner, don't say 'I hope I meet someone special', say '*I have met someone special*'. If your goal is to lose weight and your target weight is 65 kg, don't say 'I am trying to lose weight', say '*I now weigh 65 kg!*'

Rule #3 Personal

The final rule in designing goals is that they need to be personal. Instead of being generic, they should mean something to you. Don't just say 'I have a new job', say '*I have a new job that is exciting and challenging*'. A goal relating to work/life balance might include something like '*I finish work by 5 pm every day – I am home in time to enjoy bath time with my children*'. Even if these examples are not relevant to you, you can see how much more inspiring and motivating the goal becomes when it has the personal element.

Exercise

Review the goals you set in the previous exercise (page 106) and make sure that each goal is a SMART goal.

For each goal:

- Provide specific details about what you are aiming to achieve.
- Include a measurement or method for determining precisely when you have achieved your goal.
- Make sure that the goal you have set is both achievable in a general sense, and realistic for you to achieve given your overall commitment to this goal.
- Include a deadline for achieving your goal.

When you have worked through each goal and feel confident that your goals really are SMART, review them one more time. This time pay close attention to the language you have used when describing your goal.

Make sure that each goal is:

- expressed in positive, not negative, terms
- described in the present tense, as if your goal has already been achieved
- described using language that makes this goal deeply personal and meaningful for you

Adrian's story

Adrian was a busy sales executive who really loved his work. The only problem was, sometimes things got so busy that all he had time for was work and no time to do any of the other things he used to enjoy doing. He wanted to work with a coach because, although he was doing well at work and had increases in his commissions to prove it, he felt like everything else in his life was beginning to unravel. He knew he needed to make some changes but he didn't know where to start.

I asked Adrian to work through the Wheel of Life exercise. Well, did he have a flat tyre! Not only was he suffering in terms of his social and recreational life, while he worked through the exercise he realised that his health was beginning to deteriorate as a result of his long work hours. Adrian couldn't even give himself a score in the relationship segment – it had been so long since he had had time to think about being in one.

He set about creating some short-term goals and quick wins to bring his life back into balance, to pump up his Wheel of Life. He committed to a 30-minute run three times a week and walking to or from work at least twice a week. I suggested he leave his iPod at home and enjoy some silence while he exercised. Not only would this goal address his declining fitness, but it would also give him time to think and collect his thoughts about the day ahead. Adrian found that the extra clarity this gave him made it easier to prioritise at work, and as a result he was much more efficient.

(continued)

Next Adrian decided to set some short-term goals relating to his social life and recreation time. He loved going to the football but he hadn't been all season — he'd just been too busy to get around to organising it. He decided to set a goal of going to one match each fortnight, and watch the game with friends over a beer and pizza the alternate week. I asked Adrian to do a ring-around and get names and dates in his diary to make it easier to commit.

The final area Adrian knew he needed to address was relationships. Not only was he not in one, he had stopped meeting new people, so there wasn't even a new relationship on the horizon. Adrian knew he needed to set a goal of creating opportunities to meet new people. Combining his interests with a social activity, he decided to join a wine-tasting club. Not only was he bound to meet new people, it would force him to leave work on time!

By putting in place these simple, effective and fun quick wins and short-term goals, Adrian was able to continue to enjoy his job while getting back to loving his life.

ARE YOUR GOALS ATTRACTIVE?

One of the major reasons people fail to achieve their goals is that they don't ensure that the goal is attractive on a personal level. They waste their goal-setting energies on things they think they should do — things they thought they *needed* to do, but didn't feel *inspired* to achieve.

I know plenty of men and women who have set exercise goals they have failed to achieve, only to find that with their impending wedding date, they become gym junkies. What happened was that they finally tapped into a way to make their goal attractive. And what can be more attractive than a desire to look your very best on your special day?

I am sure you can all recall something you set out to do in the past and failed. It might not have 'officially' been a goal, but when you look back later you realise that you never really wanted to make it happen. By having hidden negative attitudes, or for that matter anything less than positive attitudes towards your goal, you are allowing your subconscious to begin sabotaging your efforts right from the start.

In my early twenties I was a smoker — I really can't believe it now — but I was…uuggh! Anyway, I made several half-hearted attempts to quit, but the truth was, I enjoyed it. I knew it was bad for me, that it was damaging my lungs and I really did think that I 'should' stop, but somehow I just didn't. One day, I finally discovered what I needed to make quitting smoking an attractive goal. I found some small, faint wrinkles! Now you might call it vanity, but there was no way I wanted to succumb to premature ageing. I set a date of two weeks' time and from that day forward I simply stated 'I am a non-smoker' and I never had another cigarette. Every time I was tempted I just had to remind myself about premature ageing and my resolve was strengthened like steel.

That was more than 12 years ago and I've never had another cigarette. So you can see, I know personally how powerful it can be to identify what is attractive to *you* about your goal.

With each goal you set, it's important to identify and engage with what makes that goal attractive to *you*. Some people even go as far as to say that the A in SMART should stand for Attractive, it is that important.

By making sure that the goals you choose to set are goals that really matter to you, you will make achieving them something you can do with ease.

BUILDING BLOCKS FOR THE LIFE OF YOUR DREAMS

Now that you have created a vision for your future, you can begin designing the goals you will need to achieve if you are to make that vision a reality. These goals will become the building blocks of your dream life.

By breaking your vision down into key elements and setting goals around those elements, you will see exactly what you need to do. Once you have designed your SMART goals, you need to determine how long it is going to take you to achieve them. It's likely that some of your goals will be medium- and long-term, so break them down into the smaller 'sub' goals you will need to achieve along the way. Every long-term goal can be broken into a series of medium-term goals and every medium-term goal can be broken down into a set of short-term goals.

Each time you find yourself thinking that a goal is out of reach or difficult to achieve, break it down into smaller goals. Have you heard the expression 'How do you eat an elephant? Piece by piece'? Well, that is exactly what we are trying to achieve here by turning your big vision into small, bite-sized pieces. Don't worry if you haven't covered every single step yet, just make sure that you are able to identify enough steps to make your vision seem like a very real future outcome.

You might find that in order to break down some of the key areas, you need to do some research, or speak to people with more experience than you about exactly what steps you need to take to make your goals happen. On the other hand, you might find that for some key elements of your vision, there is no right or wrong way to make them a reality and it's simply about choosing where to begin, setting a goal and working towards making it happen.

Having a vision is powerful, but without designing the goals you need to achieve to make it happen, you run the risk that your vision will remain a dream – about how your life could be.

Exercise

Now it's time to use what you have learnt about goal-setting to create the building blocks for the life of your dreams.

Using your vision statement, work through the key elements and design a master goal for each one. At this stage, you don't need to focus on the medium- or short-term goals required to get there, just concentrate on the big picture. Make sure you express your goals as positive, present tense, personal goals that are SMART.

You might find that you have already designed some of these master or vision goals in the previous exercises. If so, revise the goals you have already set, to make sure they are 100 per cent consistent with your vision for the future.

When you have completed this exercise you will have a very clear idea of what you need to do if you are to create the life of your dreams.

KEEP IT SMALL AND SIMPLE

I cannot stress enough the importance of designing your goals so that they are small and simple. You want to set yourself up for success, not failure, so the simpler and easier to achieve they are, the better.

When it was time to dream, I encouraged you to 'dream big' and while you were creating your vision, you had every encouragement to make it as bold as you wanted, but believe it or not, the key to achieving this big, bold future is to make sure that your goals are small and simple.

You want to make it as easy as possible to make progress towards your dream life. I'm not saying that some of your goals can't be exciting or challenge you, but make sure you know the small and simple steps needed to achieve this exciting and challenging outcome.

Occasionally you might find you have broken your goals down into too many steps – as if, in order to keep things small and simple, you have inadvertently created nothing but a big to-do list! When this happens, put your list aside for the moment and focus on the bigger picture. Don't throw it out. All you have done is create a head-start with the information you will need when it's time to move on to planning. You're simply ahead of schedule!

Exercise

Continuing on from the previous exercise (page 110), I want you to start breaking your big-picture goals into smaller, more achievable steps:

- Start with one of your vision or master goals.
- Break that goal down into the two or three long-term goals needed to achieve your vision.
- Then break each long-term goal into two or three medium-term goals.
- Break each medium-term goal into two or three short-term goals.
- Finally, see if you can break each short-term goal into a couple of quick wins you can implement straight away.

You might want to work through this goal-setting exercise using a whiteboard, or use colour-coded note cards or Post-it® notes. Different colours can indicate short-, medium- or long-term goals. It helps if you can stick your cards or Post-its on a wall or large table so you can see how your future is mapping out.

Don't worry if you can't come up with every single goal you need to achieve. As you begin to achieve these goals, what you need to work on next will become apparent.

When you have come up with the majority of the goals you need to create the life of your dreams, write them in your journal. Dedicate at least one page to each key vision element. Make sure that the goals you write down are positive, present tense, personal SMART goals.

GOAL-SETTING AND GOAL-GETTING

Setting goals is important, but achieving those goals is even more important. Building a detailed plan of action is covered in the next chapter, but for now I want to share with you my top-five rules for achieving your goals. After all, writing down your goals is just one step along the road to achieving them.

> **Setting goals is important, but achieving those goals is even more important.**

Rule #1 Write them down and read them regularly

I can't tell you enough times how important it is to write your goals down, but equally important is that you read over your goal list regularly, at least every morning and night. You want to make working towards those goals seem like the most natural thing in the world and the best way to do that is to make them part of your world.

Rule #2 Don't share your goals with anyone and everyone

It can be so exciting when you start experiencing the power of goal-setting that you find yourself wanting to tell the world. Don't! Keep your goals close to your chest. Share them with two or three people you know you can count on to provide unconditional support. You don't want to give people the opportunity to inadvertently or intentionally undermine your goals or your progress because of their own limiting beliefs.

Rule #3 The rule of threes

Don't work on too many of your goals all at once. Although you might have many goals within your overall focus, it's most effective to limit yourself to working toward just three goals in each category at any one time; three short-term, three medium- and three long-term goals. As you achieve your goals in each category you can begin to incorporate other goals into your schedule. Don't worry if this seems limiting. The narrower your focus, the more you will achieve over time.

Rule #4 Review your progress

As you work towards achieving your goals, it's important to keep track of your progress. Not only will this help you acknowledge how far you have come, but it will also help you to learn from your own experience. Have a weekly review of your short-term goals, a monthly review of your medium-term goals and an annual review of your long-term goals.

Rule #5 Celebrate your success

It is important that you remember to celebrate each small goal you achieve along the way to your long-term goals. The more you celebrate your success, the more you will feel successful, the more you will become successful – so get celebrating!

Exercise

In addition to your regular journal I suggest you create a special journal specifically to monitor your progress with your goals. Some people turn their regular journal over and work from the back, or if your journal is in the form of a file, you might want to create a separate section for mapping the progress of each goal. Include a copy of your vision statement at the start of your goals journal.

Next include a page for each vision goal and behind that a page for each goal that will contribute to the achievement of your vision. Use these pages to make notes and monitor your progress. Review your goals journal daily, making a note of the things you have done that day which have taken you one step closer to living the life you've always dreamed of.

You can use goal cards for inspiration when you are on the move or away from your journal. Using an index card the size of a large business card, write down the top three goals you are working on. On the other side of the card write down three affirmations or positive statements that will support you as you achieve your goals.

Look at your goal card regularly throughout the day. One idea is to keep it in your wallet as a reminder of your goals every time you go to spend money!

Although one goal card could last you quite a while it's advisable to create a new card each week to keep your goals fresh in your mind.

THERE IS NO SUCH THING AS FAILURE

It can be hard to know how long it will take to achieve your goals. Sometimes when we set the time scale on our goals, we are being naively ambitious; unable to anticipate hiccups or problems along the way.

Whatever the reason, if you find you have not achieved your goal in the time frame you have set, remember one thing – you have *not* failed. All you are experiencing is what I call the timing difference between effort and reward!

Remember, you are not psychic, you can't see into the future. All you can do is make the best possible estimation based on the information you have available. You might find you need to review the goal and look at ways to make it more realistic or achievable, or you need to work harder than you had realised, or maybe you just need to approach it in a different way.

Whatever the reason, as long as you have tried, just because you haven't yet achieved your goal, it doesn't mean you have failed

Remember, you are so much closer to your goal than you were when you began. Don't use a setback like this as an excuse to give up. Keep things in perspective by remembering that all you are experiencing is a little timing delay and as long as you maintain your commitment, you will definitely get to your goal.

Tamara's story

Tamara had resigned from her job as a marketing manager when her son was born, but now that he had started pre-school she was looking for a part-time job; one that used her marketing skills, but was not as demanding as her priorities had changed. She was well aware such jobs were rarely advertised and didn't

(continued)

know quite how to go about getting one, so she decided to work with a coach.

Tamara and I agreed that she would need to take a 'creative' approach to finding a job and since very few quality part-time jobs are advertised, the best job-searching strategy would be through the 'hidden' job market – planning, research and networking.

She set a goal of being back in the paid workforce in six months' time. Over the next five months she was diligent in doing everything required to source an exciting new job, but as her deadline came close nothing was on the horizon. She had attended networking events and let her wider social circle know what she was looking for, and she had met people for countless conversations, coffees and lunches.

When I spoke to Tamara the week before her deadline she was feeling dejected. She couldn't work out what she was doing wrong and why she was almost certainly not going to achieve her goal. I reminded her that even if she didn't have a new job by the end of the following week she hadn't failed – she simply hadn't succeeded yet! Her deadline of six months was a self-created deadline, put into place to motivate her into action and keep her committed. All she could control was the effort she made, not the decisions other people needed to make.

I encouraged her to remain positive and not to give up hope – success was surely just around the corner. And I was right. By the end of the seventh month Tamara had been offered four jobs. Her only challenge then was deciding which one to take!

SET YOUR SAILS OR DECIDE TO DRIFT

People sometimes say to me, 'I don't know if I want to set goals, maybe I just want to see what opportunities come my way.' My answer to that is always – no problem! Deciding not to set goals is a perfectly acceptable approach if you are not looking to achieve a specific outcome. But if you do know what you want, setting goals will actively help you to create opportunities that will bring you closer to your desired result.

No one can force you to take up every opportunity that comes along. You will still be able to pick and choose as you create your future. But if you are working with a specific set of goals, you will be able to see more clearly which opportunities are taking you closer to or further from the life of your dreams.

There is absolutely nothing wrong with just seeing which way the wind blows, as long as you ensure this is a conscious decision. What I don't recommend is choosing to drift, hoping you will end up at your desired destination. If you do know where you want to be, goal-setting is by far the best way to set and follow a course to the life of your dreams.

KEY LESSONS – DESIGNING REAL AND SPECIFIC GOALS

1. If you want to create powerful goals, make sure they are SMART – specific, measurable, achievable, realistic and time-based.

2. If every goal you set is positive, in the present tense and personal you will soon start to feel that achieving that goal is the most natural outcome in the world.

3. Make a dramatic improvement in your everyday life by finding some quick wins and short-term goals you can achieve easily if you put your mind to it.

4. Your dreams should be exciting and your vision should be bold, but if you want to achieve your goals, they need to be small and simple.

5. Don't set goals for what you think you 'should' do. If you focus on what is truly attractive to you, your goals will be much easier to achieve.

6. By designing goals based on the key elements of your vision, you will ensure that your vision soon becomes a reality.

7. To make sure you achieve your goals:
   - Write them down.
   - Keep them private.
   - Focus on no more than three goals at once.
   - Review your progress.
   - Celebrate your success.

8. Sometimes there can be a timing difference between effort and reward. If you don't achieve your goals in the time frame you have set, never give up. Success is always just around the corner!

CHAPTER 6
Developing unshakeable self-confidence

Whatever your vision for the future involves, increasing your confidence and building your self-esteem are essential if you want to create the life of your dreams. Perhaps one of the keys to your vision is unlimited self-confidence and the courage to undertake anything you dream. Or you simply might want to become a more confident person. You might have identified building your self-confidence as an important step in being able to achieve the other goals that will bring you *real* success and happiness.

Even if you already feel you are a confident person, you can still build on that confidence. If you invest your energy in building unshakeable confidence, you will know that nothing can ever knock you down or take the wind out of your sails.

Whatever goals you have set for yourself, it is always just as important to work on *who* you want to be, as it is to work on *what* you want to achieve. Building resilient self-confidence is an essential part of being the best you can be.

Remember that it takes courage and commitment to create the life of your dreams. At any point you could choose an easier path and live a pleasant but ordinary life. There is nothing wrong with that at all, but if you want your dreams to come true – and a future that is filled with *real* success and happiness – then you most likely need to work on *who* you are in addition to *what* you need to do.

Unshakeable self-confidence is not about never having a bad day. We all have days when our confidence receives a bump or a knock and we wish we had stayed in bed! But if your confidence levels are unwavering, then these incidences have no impact at the core of your self-belief.

Having unshakeable self-confidence is not about being invincible, it's about how quickly you can dust yourself off after a disappointment and get your confidence levels back on track.

Think of an old oak tree. Things may come along that rustle its leaves or snap off a branch but it is virtually impossible to do any serious damage to the trunk – an oak tree is truly unshakeable. That's the level of resilience you want to build for your confidence level and self-esteem.

Having unshakeable self-confidence is not about being invincible, it's about how quickly you can dust yourself off after a disappointment.

Developing unlimited self-confidence is a choice. While some people may have naturally higher levels of confidence than others, you can consciously choose to build up your own confidence.

BELIEVE IN YOURSELF

It is one thing to have confidence in something you know you're good at – like being confident in your job when you have just received an excellent performance appraisal, or confidence in your ability to achieve financial success because you saved a sum of money. In both of these examples, your confidence is based on some proof of your ability in a specific subject or area. I call this 'subject-based confidence' – a belief in your ability to do something because you know you can do it. All subject-based confidence is highly valuable, but because it is based on what you can do, not who you are, it is easily threatened by external factors – a boss you disagree with or an unforeseen expense that drains your savings.

True self-belief comes from an innate confidence. A confidence in who you are, not just what you can do. Innate confidence is about having a fundamental belief that you will have everything you need, achieve everything you want and have the best possible life. Innate confidence is about truly believing in yourself, without justification, simply because you are you. It is not dependent on external factors, by its very nature it is invulnerable to external influences. It is about believing in yourself, your character, your strengths and knowing that as long as you focus on being the best you can be, everything will turn out well for you.

Innate confidence is about having a fundamental belief that you will have everything you need, achieve everything you want and have the best possible life.

Exercise

It's time to do an audit on your confidence and sense of self-belief. First, I want you to give your current overall confidence level a score out of ten, where ten is the highest mark. Then I want you to make a note of the things that need to change if your confidence level was to move from its current score to a 9.5/10. What would you need to change about the way you think or act? Aim to have at least three items on this list.

Next, make a list of six specific areas in which your confidence is strong, say above 6.5/10.

Finally, I want you to make a list of six specific areas in which your confidence levels are low. For each item on your list, make a note of one thing you could do to make an improvement in that particular area.

You will find this audit worth completing on a regular basis, say every six to twelve months, to keep track of how your confidence levels are increasing over time.

Although innate confidence is not based on what you know, it can be developed by working to overcome your limiting beliefs and constantly replacing any negative thoughts with positive ones. If you focus on these simple but powerful tasks, innate confidence will soon become a natural part of who you are.

ARE YOU A HIGH ACHIEVER OR AN OVER-ACHIEVER?

Since you are reading this book I am assuming that achieving the things you set out to do is an appealing idea, but the question is, are you a high achiever or an over-achiever – and do you know the difference?

Over-achiever

An over-achiever is always working on several things at once, doing everything they can to prove their value. They are perfectionists who won't stop until they can guarantee they have achieved 100 per cent of whatever they are trying to do. An over-achiever has a hard time saying no and often takes on too much, then feels deeply resentful at being overloaded.

Over-achievers are often highly competitive, always measuring themselves against others, never content to simply rely on achieving their personal best. They rarely give themselves compliments, instead relying on feedback from others to let them know whether their efforts were sufficient. Criticism hurts them deeply and they are quick to dismiss any compliments they receive.

Perfectionist is just another word for over-achiever. Perfectionism is a trap – as long as you try to be perfect, you'll never be good enough!

Over-achievement is a symptom of vulnerable self-esteem. Deep down, over-achievers are worried that nothing they do is ever good enough.

High achiever

On the surface, a high achiever may appear similar to an over-achiever. A high achiever, by the very nature of the term, is someone who regularly appears to be in the process of achieving something, but there are some fundamental differences.

A high achiever is able to measure their performance against the goals they have set for themselves. They are not waiting for approval from anyone. A high achiever has a robust self-esteem. They always give their best and know their best is good enough.

Notice I have used the words 'vulnerable' and 'robust' when referring to self-esteem, not 'high' and 'low'. While some over-achievers do have low self-esteem, quite often it is simply that their self-esteem is vulnerable, rather than unshakeable.

YOUR MOST IMPORTANT CONVERSATION IS WITH YOURSELF

Does every internal conversation you have work towards building, or eroding, your belief in yourself?

If you are working towards developing a greater level of confidence in yourself one of the most important things you can do is pay attention to your inner dialogue. To build unshakeable self-confidence, you really do need to focus on becoming your own biggest fan.

Constantly listen to your inner dialogue. Make sure that the messages you are sending your subconscious consistently work towards building your confidence rather than slowly breaking it down piece by piece.

It is important to listen to the messages about the areas in which you are working to build confidence, and it's also important to listen to the dialogue you are engaged in about your confidence levels in general. There is no point working on affirmations designed to build your confidence in a particular area if you are not working to build unshakeable confidence in who you are at the same time. You need to make sure that every internal conversation you have is a positive one, and one that ultimately supports you as you create the life of your dreams.

Constantly listen to your inner dialogue.

Review the list of affirmations you created in Chapter 3 and see if you need to add some additional messages to reform your thoughts about areas in which you would like to be confident, or your confidence levels in general.

You might want to try:

- 'I am a confident and intelligent person.'
- 'I radiate confidence.'
- 'I believe in myself unconditionally. Others believe in me too.'

Exercise

Spend a couple of days paying extra attention to your inner dialogue. Make a note of every time you engage in any internal conversations that undermine your confidence and self-belief. There's no need to write down exact details of your negative thoughts, in fact, it's better if you don't capture all the gory details! Just make a note of any general thoughts preventing you from having unshakeable self-confidence.

For each negative thought you capture, I want you to write down an affirmation or positive statement you can use to reform your thoughts. I also want you to make a note if something you were doing or experiencing triggered your negative self-talk. This might occur:

- When you see someone who is attractive, you have negative thoughts about your own appearance.
- When you hear about a friend's success at work, you find yourself in an internal conversation filled with doubts about your own professional abilities.
- When you are trying something new for the first time.
- If you are finding the goals you have set for yourself to be tougher than expected.

It is just as important to capture *when* you have negative internal conversations as it is to capture *what* you say. If you know which activities and experiences are most likely to trigger self-doubt, you will be able to prepare for these times by concentrating on thoughts that build your self-belief and confidence.

PLAY TO YOUR STRENGTHS

In this day and age, we are all so focused on improving ourselves that we forget to celebrate who we are and our existing positive qualities and strengths. So often I hear people say, 'I have so much to improve,' or 'I need to work on so many things,' without taking a moment to acknowledge what they already do well.

We are all so focused on improving ourselves that we forget to celebrate who we are and our existing positive qualities and strengths.

It's so much easier to focus on our faults, flaws or negative qualities. While it is important to work on these *learning opportunities,* it's equally important to focus on our strengths and positive qualities. It's vital to accept yourself for who you are. Any improvements you are making to yourself should be a positive experience, one that builds your confidence, not a negative experience that only serves to erode your self-belief and hold you back in life. You will find your confidence levels steadily diminish if you focus on all the things you could be changing, instead of focusing on all the things you should be celebrating.

There is a popular expression that says you should work *in* your strengths and *on* your weaknesses. What this means is that you should concentrate your attention on your positive qualities and make sure that the choices you make in life put your strengths to good use. At the same time, make sure that you are also focusing on one or two of your areas for improvement so that over time you start to become the best you can be.

A crucial part of building unshakeable self-confidence is accepting who you are and knowing what is special about *you*. You already have a lot going for you, so when you think about improving yourself, make sure you recognise how wonderful you already are.

Exercise

One of the most powerful tools for building unshakeable self-confidence is to acknowledge all your strengths and positive qualities. Most people find it easy to write a list of their weaknesses, but much harder to focus on their strengths.

Complete the following lists and watch your self-confidence soar:

1. List the 10 things in your life you are most proud of.
2. List 10 things you are good at.
3. List 10 of your character strengths.
4. List your 10 most attractive qualities. Note you can include both internal and external qualities in this list.

Don't worry if you can't complete the full 10 items for each list on your first attempt. Review your lists regularly and keep adding to them over time until each list includes at least 10 items. And when you have completed the first 10, I want you to start working on the next 10!

Keep this list in your journal. Reading through it will give your self-confidence a big boost, so refer to it whenever you are feeling down or your confidence levels are not as high as they could be.

LIFE IS NOT A COMPETITION

So many people move through life constantly striving to be better than the next person, treating everything they do as if it were a competition – one in which there is only one winner and everyone else must be a loser.

What these people don't realise is that by treating everything as a contest, continually pitting themselves against others, they are slowly eroding their confidence and self-esteem. After all, it's impossible to win all the time. Even the world's greatest athletes have known some bitter defeats.

As long as your confidence and sense of self-worth is based on a comparison, you will always be in a losing situation.

It is far more desirable and sustainable to view life as an *experience*, not a competition. Sometimes you'll come out on top, but other times, while you won't have 'won', you will have learnt so much that it will be of far greater value than any straightforward victory.

If you want to build unshakeable confidence, you need to commit to being the best that you can be. There is no winning; there will always be someone with more and, of course, always someone with less. Each of these comparisons fails to take into account the whole story. The richer person might be lonely, the poorer man might have love in his life that money could never buy. It is the same for any other comparison you can think of. Whichever way you twist it, there is just no winning in life if you play by those rules.

Don't worry, I'm not suggesting you concede defeat! All I want you to do is change the rules of the game. The only competition you need to be in is with yourself, and the only thing you measure yourself against is your personal best and the personal goals you have set. As long as you work towards being the best you can be, you will always be a winner!

John's story

John always believed that he was a high achiever. An excellent sportsman with a burgeoning career in the legal profession, he was used to being the best at whatever he did. But lately he had found himself feeling worried about his future and deeply stressed whenever he had to make a significant decision.

When John began to examine his inner dialogue, he found that he was highly critical of himself and others. Somewhere along the line he had fallen into the pattern of being an over-achiever. He was continually taking on more work than he could really manage and constantly worrying that nothing he did was ever good enough.

He had developed the negative habit of comparing himself with everyone around him and had become highly critical of his own performance. By constantly measuring his progress against that of everyone else, John no longer knew what his best was, and he certainly didn't know if it was good enough.

I reminded him that he was an intelligent and highly capable man. I asked him to stop worrying about constantly doing the right thing and explained that by redeveloping his trust in himself

(continued)

he would be giving his confidence a big boost. At the same time I asked him to pay attention to his inner dialogue and to take note of each time he found himself 'benchmarking' himself against other people, and to replace that thought with an affirmation about his own abilities.

John hadn't realised he had fallen into the trap of over-achievement. By concentrating on achieving his personal best he was able to break this habit and go back to being the confident high achiever he truly was.

STEP OUTSIDE YOUR COMFORT ZONE

One of the best ways to build unshakeable confidence is to step outside your comfort zone – regularly! Stepping outside your comfort zone is like giving your sense of self a shake-up. It's easy to become complacent: I'm good at this, I'm not good at that. But how do you really know what you're capable of if you never try?

You don't want to place yourself in a position where you might lose everything you have, or injury yourself terribly, but at the same time a life in which you are completely safe and nothing ever challenges you or makes you uncomfortable is unlikely to provide you with *real* success and happiness. Think of it as taking safe risks.

When you hear the saying 'Do one thing each day that scares you', the idea is not to be afraid for your safety and well being. Instead we are talking about things that scare you in an emotional sense – things that place you at risk of failure or disappointment, but at the same time take you one step closer to your dreams.

Stepping outside your comfort zone is like giving your sense of self a shake-up.

You might think that you're not good at public speaking, but in fact you have never stood up and spoken before a group before. If you step outside your comfort zone and just attempt this, regardless of the outcome, your confidence will receive a huge boost – simply because you tried!

When I am about to attempt something outside my comfort zone I feel terrified and excited at the same time. I can literally feel it in the pit of my stomach, but I don't let that stop me! Whenever I have this feeling, I treat it as a good sign. After all, any experience that can create such a strong response must really be important in my life and is definitely worth going for.

Every time you step out of your comfort zone you send a message to your subconscious that says, 'I wasn't afraid to try.' Your subconscious receives this message as a sign of self-belief, and your confidence levels will increase accordingly. The more you risk failure, the more you will believe you are a success.

Sarah's story

When Sarah returned to work after her youngest child started school, she began an entirely new career as a sales rep. Although she was highly confident in her abilities as a mother, her confidence in herself as a professional woman was somewhat fragile. Intellectually she knew she had the skills and commitment to do well, but believing in herself 100 per cent was something else all together.

While Sarah was excellent at relationship building, she was deeply shy when it came to meeting people for the first time and speaking in public was something that made her feel sick. She knew she would have to overcome this shyness to achieve her potential in this next stage of her life.

During her first few coaching sessions she learned to overcome her limiting beliefs and to develop affirmations or positive beliefs that would support her in building confidence. I asked her to heighten her awareness, or 'catch herself', when she put herself down and then to replace those negative thoughts with a positive statement affirming her abilities and desire to succeed.

Sarah began to focus, not on the fact that some things in life were difficult, but on how good she would feel when she had done them anyway – be that walking up to a crowd of people she hadn't already met or taking the lead in her team meetings.

By regularly stepping out of her comfort zone, and using affirmations to build her self-belief, Sarah has become a more confident person; one who does not let self-doubt get in her way.

(continued)

When she meets someone new, they find her to be a confident and outgoing person. Keen to continue receiving the benefits of stepping outside her comfort zone, Sarah is also planning to give a presentation to 400 people at her next industry conference.

Exercise

It's essential to step outside your comfort zone regularly if you want to build unshakeable self-confidence. Doing one thing each day that scares you, can be quite overwhelming, so make a list of 12 things you can do over the next 12 months that feel scary now, but that you know will give your confidence a big boost when you do them. It doesn't matter if the items on your list are big or small, what matters is that they are taking you out of your comfort zone.

If you aim to do one thing each month that scares you, at the end of the year your confidence levels will have soared!

DETOX YOUR LIFE

One of the most important things you can do as you work to build your confidence is to eliminate negative influences in your life. You have already become practised at listening to your internal dialogue. Now I want you to start paying attention to the conversations you have with other people. While some people will be supporting you 110 per cent, others will be saying things to bring you down. Some of this negativity will be conscious, but most of it will be the subconscious result of their own limiting beliefs and the narrow vision they hold for their future.

The truth is, as you build your confidence and move closer towards the life of your dreams, not everybody will be comfortable with the progress you are making. When you find someone is responding to you in a negative or critical way, remember that it's about them, not you.

One of the most important things you can do as you work to build your confidence is to eliminate negative influences in your life.

If your vision is to have financial freedom, pay attention to how much time you spend with people who continually talk about not having enough money. Just by engaging in their conversation you will be participating in their poverty mentality.

If your goal is to quit smoking or lose weight, keep well away from 'friends' who offer you cigarettes or fattening food, just to see if you can be tempted. You want people in your life who will do anything they can to support you with your goals, not those who will subtly, or not so subtly, work against you.

If you are working towards creating the life of your dreams, watch the conversations you have with people who tell you that life wasn't meant to be easy, or that you are being unrealistic. Remember, you don't need to waste your energy explaining to them that you create your own reality. They can learn that lesson in their own time, if and when they choose to do so.

When I began to redesign my future, detoxing my life had an enormous impact. Suddenly, whenever I was in a conversation, it was as if I had developed supersonic hearing. I could hear what was *really* being said. I discovered who in my extended circle was worrying incessantly; who spoke of never having enough money even though they had a six-figure income; and who made jokes at other people's expense or put their friends down.

In most cases it was easy to spend less, if any, time with the people concerned. I also discovered that the company of some people was so toxic that I chose never to spend time in their company again.

Unfortunately it isn't always that easy. If the toxic influence is a family member or someone you love dearly, you will still want to spend some time with them. Instead of adopting a drastic approach, simply be vigilant about which conversations you engage in when you are with them. The last thing you need is to be constantly defending your goals and justifying your vision. There is no need to quit their company altogether, just keep your conversations simple and superficial – things like films you have seen and books you have read.

Another major toxic influence in your life is worry, a subconscious endorsement of your fears that serves to subtly undermine your confidence. It's hard for your confidence to thrive when you are living in fear. I firmly believe that there is no value in worrying whatsoever. Either things are within your control, or they're not. If there are aspects of your life that are causing concern, make a plan to do something about them. Conquering your worries will give your confidence a big boost.

And if you are worrying about things that are beyond your control, I have one word of advice – *stop*! Worrying about them is simply an indulgence and I know I'd prefer to indulge in chocolate over worry any day!

Exercise

Eliminating the negative influences in your life is not only important in building your confidence levels, it's also deeply empowering as you start saying 'This is no longer acceptable in my life' – to things that have been wearing you down.

Make a list of ten ways that you can 'detox' your life. Include your own habits and behaviours as well as those of the people around you.

Don't worry, I won't ask you to go 'cold turkey' on all of the negative influences in your life – although of course you can if you want to! Instead I want you to make a note next to each item, of the date that you intend to say goodbye to that particular negativity for once and for all.

TRUST YOURSELF TO MAKE THE RIGHT DECISION

One of the best ways to build your confidence is to trust in yourself a little more. This may sound like a catch-22 – how can you trust in yourself if you lack confidence? – but sometimes you need to take a leap of faith.

Life is filled with choices and it takes courage to make a decision, rather than just drift along. Some people feel that before they can make a decision they need to canvass all their friends and loved ones for their opinions to ensure that they make the right decision. They mistakenly believe that calling on the support of others in this way is a sign of strength and wisdom.

Calling on the support of others can be a sign of strength, but not when you are using it as a way of eliminating the fear of getting something wrong, as a way of outsourcing your decision-making to others.

There are no guarantees in life and it is a mistake to feel that by getting everyone else's input you are reducing the risk of getting something wrong. In actual fact, you are compounding the situation – the more you listen to others, the less you are able to listen to yourself and trust your instincts as to what is the right answer for you.

The more self-sufficient you become and the more you can trust in yourself and be strong in your decisions, the more your confidence will increase. Remember, there are no right or wrong decisions. As long as you knowingly and consciously make a decision, it will always be the right one for you. In the end, all we can do any time we make a decision is make it based on the best available information.

Life is filled with choices and it takes courage to make a decision, rather than just drift along.

Of course, as time goes on, more information may come to hand that indicates that another alternative may have been a better one. But unless you could see into the future and consciously ignored this fact, your decision is still the best one.

Make sure you are not living in fear of regret. As long as you trust in yourself and consciously make decisions, you will always make the right decision. So what if, with the wisdom of hindsight, you might have done something differently? With the wisdom of hindsight, there are a lot of things I might have done differently, but unless someone is selling hindsight lenses for my sunglasses, those experiences will remain things that I have been able to learn from, not things that I regret!

WHO ARE YOU NOT TO SHINE?

One question clients raise again and again is their fear of becoming 'overconfident'. Although their confidence levels might need improving, they are worried about appearing arrogant, overbearing and intimidating.

Authentic confidence is never arrogant or overbearing. Real confidence is not about being better than someone else — it's about knowing you are the best *you* can be. When your confidence is authentic, not only does it radiate from you like a brilliant golden glow, it actually lifts others up and sweeps them along in your brilliance.

If you think of someone you know who appears overconfident or arrogant, ask yourself what they are afraid of, or making up for. Overconfidence or arrogance is a symptom of fear and inadequacy. At some level people who are arrogant or overconfident are making up for a deep, ingrained fear that they really aren't good enough at all.

As long as the confidence you are developing is honest and pure and based on a recognition that you are a unique individual who is proud of always being the best you can be, other people won't be put off. Instead, they will find your presence encouraging and inspiring.

KEY LESSONS – BUILDING UNSHAKEABLE SELF-CONFIDENCE

1. Innate confidence is about being confident in who you are, not just what you can do. It is about developing a deep sense of self-belief.

2. Be a high achiever, not an over-achiever. Know that as long as you give your best, it will always be good enough.

3. Become your own biggest fan. Make sure that every internal conversation you have works towards building your confidence and self-belief.

4. When you think about improving yourself, make sure you remember all your positive qualities. Accept yourself and acknowledge how special you already are.

5. Life is an experience, not a competition. If the only person you ever compete against is yourself, you will always be a winner.

6. Don't be afraid to try. Stepping outside your comfort zone sends a strong message to your subconscious that you believe in yourself and your confidence levels will automatically rise.

7. Eliminate negative influences from your life. Pay attention to the negative conversations you have with yourself and other people. They are slowly eroding your confidence.

8. There are no right or wrong decisions. As long as you consciously make a decision, it will always be the right one for you!

CHAPTER 7
Building a detailed plan of action

By now you will have developed a clear idea of what your dream life looks like, you will have your goals and you have begun working on who you need to become if you are to achieve *real* success and happiness in your life.

It's now time to start working on the detail – the specifics of what you need to accomplish to create the life of your dreams. It's time to formulate a plan, and not just any plan, a plan of action: a plan that will both compel and inspire you into action!

A lot of people are overwhelmed by the idea of planning, but a plan is simply a list of things to do including the date by which each item needs to be completed. If you take some time to carefully construct and word your plan, it will be like an affirmation in motion, a confirmatory message to your subconscious that you can and will make every part of your plan a reality.

You deserve to have the life of your dreams and a plan of action is a step-by-step account of what you need to do to make your dream a reality.

YOU NEED A MAP FOR YOUR JOURNEY

Even though you might have heard the expression 'to fail to plan is to plan to fail', you might still feel like skipping this chapter and not bothering with planning at all. Would you still be able to create the life of your dreams? Perhaps...

Plenty of wonderful things can happen in this life as a result of luck, of being in the right place at the right time. But if your goal is to create financial freedom, would you really just buy a lottery ticket and sit back and wait for your numbers to come up? If you truly want to create financial freedom, by all means buy that lottery ticket, in fact, buy one every week, but by creating a savings and investment plan the odds that you will create financial freedom are looking a lot better than 1 in 15 million!

The bigger your dream the more important it is to have a plan, but you can also use planning to achieve the simplest of goals. Who hasn't found themselves in a situation where they have had something on their mental 'to-do' list for what seems like forever, and still never find the time to get it done. With a plan, you have a clear idea of what can be done and by when, which makes it much easier to make things happen.

Unless you can see into the future, having a plan won't guarantee results, but it will increase the likelihood that you will get to where you want to go, in the shortest possible time, with the fewest of deviations.

Just as a road map tells you when to turn right, when to turn left and helps you find your way back if you are off track, a plan will help you to determine what to do first, what to do next and let you know which things are interdependent. A plan will let you know if you are on track, ahead of schedule or in desperate need of a shortcut!

Not only will a plan tell you what to do and when to do it, it will also help you determine how long it is likely to take, to achieve each of the goals along the way to your destination — your dream life.

Will having a plan make me boring?

Some people worry that having a plan will make their life seem dull, or take the spontaneity out of things. This is a perfectly reasonable concern — until you understand how a plan can really affect your life.

There are a couple of ways to think about this. First, what is more boring — having a plan that shows you how to achieve your ideal future, or never making your ideal future a reality? I know which option I'd choose!

But that doesn't adequately address the question. Will having a plan make me one of *those* boring people who always know what is going to happen and when? Will I become one of those people who have no time for adventure or variety in their life, who live every minute according to a timetable.

Well, let me reassure you. I am assuming that because you are reading this book you are interested in the idea of creating a life you really love and that means you are not a boring person! What makes someone appear boring is a lack of inspiration in their life and a lack of spirit in the way they choose to live it.

The very fact that you have chosen to work towards creating the life of your dreams means you are the kind of person who couldn't be boring if you tried. And no plan of action has the power to change that!

There's another, equally fundamental, reason why having a plan won't make your life dull. Knowing what you need to do, when you need to do it, will free up so much of the energy you previously spent worrying about how your life was going to turn out, and wondering if you were making the right decisions about your future. You will find you now have so much spare energy that your life will be more dynamic than ever.

As you observe yourself achieving your goals and see yourself growing closer and closer to your vision for your future, your life will feel so exciting, and you will be so busy planning the next step that you won't be able to remember why you were ever concerned.

Carla's story

Carla had always known that planning was essential. As a business development manager for a major pharmaceutical company she was familiar with business plans, marketing plans and her various sales targets. But when it came to creating plans for her personal success she was deeply resistant.

Initially she wasn't sure of the reason behind her resistance, but after several coaching sessions she finally confessed that she was worried she would become 'one of those *boring* people' if she started to work to a plan. We spent some time discussing what Carla wanted out of life and it soon became clear that she had big ambitions, not just for her working life, but also for her personal life. I asked her to experiment with the idea of planning. She was welcome to drop it if she felt she was becoming too 'boring', but in the meantime I wanted her to see just how much she could achieve if she worked to a plan.

(continued)

Carla was surprised to discover that she *loved* working to a plan. It suited her ambitions perfectly as she was able to see herself growing closer and closer, step by step, to the life of her dreams. She found that when she worked to a plan she stopped worrying about her future, because she could see how she would achieve her goals over time.

Not only was working to a plan never boring, Carla soon found she was so inspired and had so much energy that her life was more exciting than ever!

Exercise

You can learn so much from your own experiences, not by criticising yourself, but by asking yourself the question, 'What would I do differently next time?'

I want you to think back through your life at some of the things you have wanted to achieve. Are there times when you would have benefited from having a plan? Or perhaps there are times when you did have a plan, but forgot to use it?

Think about the things you have tried to achieve in the past and make notes about what you would do differently if you were to attempt to achieve those goals again.

PLANNING 101

As I have already mentioned, at its simplest, a plan is a to-do list with dates. So, are you ready to create a to-do list with dates that leads you to the life of your dreams?

One of the easiest ways to create a plan is to work with a list of threes.

Choose one of your goals. Break down that goal into the three key steps required to achieve it. Now break down each of those steps into three steps, and so on, until you have broken down your goal into small, easy-to-complete steps. Next to each of these steps, make an estimation of how long it will take to achieve it.

Depending on your goal, you can either plan forwards, if the achievement date is not critical; or plan backwards, if you have a deadline you feel you just can't miss. Create a timeline for your activities to indicate what needs to happen, and by when, if you are to achieve your goal.

For those of you who like to work more visually you can do the same exercise with Post-it® notes on a wall or table. You might want to continue with the list of threes. Alternatively, you could simply brainstorm all of the activities you can think of that might be required to achieve your goal. Write down each of these activities on a separate Post-it®. Again make a note of how long you think each activity will take to complete.

Next, start arranging the Post-its® in the order you think you will need to go about the tasks. Some tasks might be must-dos whereas others might be things you would like to do. Don't forget that you can carry out some activities concurrently, while other items might be dependent on the completion of the preceding one. Don't worry if your plan isn't perfect. A plan is a guide, not something set in stone.

How you document your plan is up to you. You might like to handwrite it in a diary, journal, calendar or on poster paper, or record it in a spreadsheet or other software planning tool. How you capture your plan is nowhere near as important as the simple fact that you have one.

YOUR PORTFOLIO OF PLANS – ANNUAL, MONTHLY, WEEKLY AND DAILY

If you really want to make achieving your long-term or big-picture goals seem effortless, you don't just need a plan, you need a portfolio of plans!

You have probably heard people talk about five-year plans. What they are usually referring to is what they want to achieve in five years' time – where they would like their lives to be. It's so easy to let the hustle and bustle of everyday life get in the way of your progress, so the idea of a five-year plan is a great one. But when the life you are looking forward to is so far into the future, you also need to be able to break that plan down into much smaller, bite-sized chunks, so that you know what you need to be working on *today*.

I use a system of interlinked plans – a portfolio of plans that cover what I want to achieve in a year, what I need to achieve month-by-month, and how that will need to convert into weekly and daily action plans if I am to achieve my goal.

The plans I use work like this:

Annual plan

This plan contains a summary of my overall plan for the year and a quarter-by-quarter break-down of how I plan to achieve those annual goals. I complete the first two quarters in detail, then group quarters three and four together. I like to wait and see how the first two quarters turn out before breaking the second six months down into more detailed outlines.

For each goal I have three key steps I believe I will need to take to achieve that 'master' goal. Remember, your annual plan is not a giant to-do list! You want the information to be simple, concise, goal-style statements of what you intend to achieve. There will be plenty of opportunities to work on the detail later.

Monthly plan

Each month, I look at what I need to achieve to meet the objectives of the quarterly component of my annual plan. I create a monthly plan by breaking down those objectives into smaller and smaller pieces. I review my monthly plan at least once a week to make sure I will achieve everything that needs to be achieved.

- The key to creating a successful monthly plan is to be mindful of how much you are trying to squeeze into a single month. Think about how much time you are really going to have available that month for working on your goals.

- The purpose of your monthly plan is simply to take you one month closer to achieving the goals in your annual plan and to break down the future you are working towards into smaller, achievable steps.
- There is no need to create a monthly plan in advance for each month of the year. Creating a plan for the current month and beginning a draft version for the following month is more than enough detailed forward thinking.

Weekly plan

Each week, look at your monthly plan and ask yourself, 'What do I need to do to make sure I can achieve the goals I have set in my monthly plan?' At this stage you want to focus on the detail – individual tasks and actions that will take you closer to your overall goal.

Daily plan

A lot of people think that a daily plan is either a to-do list for the day or simply a page from their diary. Both a to-do list and a diary are important, but it is essential that each day you do two or three things that take you closer to your overall goals, and that you *prioritise* these items over the *administrivia* that can easily fill your day.

Remember, great years are achieved through a series of consistently great days.

Exercise

Go back to the detailed vision goals you created. If your goals were SMART, they would have included a deadline or other time-based information.

Begin by arranging each of your primary goals into an annual plan. Break your annual plan into quarters and assign your goals to the relevant three-monthly period. Remember the rule of threes, so in any given quarter, you don't want to be working on more than three long-term, three medium-term and three short-term goals.

Once you have arranged your goals over the coming year, focus on the next three months, or first quarter, of your plan. Start arranging your medium- and shorter-term goals, the ones that will, over time, achieve your long-term objectives.

Next, look at the coming month and break it down into all the key activities you will need to accomplish if you are going to achieve your goals. If you want to, you can complete a plan for each of the three months of the quarter, but it's also fine just to work on one month and at the end of the month, when you have achieved your goals for that month, you can then begin creating the following month's plan.

Starting from today, create a weekly plan of the key actions you will need to complete to achieve your monthly goals. You can then create a daily plan, with a focus on the tasks you will need to do to achieve your weekly goals.

> **You don't just need a plan —
> you need a portfolio of plans!**

WORKING YOUR PLAN

It's not enough just to create a plan, you have to *work* your plan. You need to review it regularly and make a conscious commitment to achieving all the elements of your plan, consistently and over time.

Many people, and for that matter businesses, spend an enormous amount of time creating the perfect plan then file it away, never to look at it again! Once you have created a plan, you need to review it constantly. You need to monitor your progress and make sure you are working your plan, and your plan is still working for you.

A plan isn't set in stone. It isn't a contract between you and the future, but rather a guide, a tool for you to use to work towards your goals. If you find that your circumstances have changed and you need to amend your plan, do it. There is nothing wrong with changing your plan, but do it consciously, don't just let it drift.

At the same time, it's important that you don't update or tweak your plan so often that it stops you from actually getting anything done!

You might want to read your *plan* daily, although because you are already reading your *goals* daily, this might not be necessary. Whatever you decide, if you want to review/revise or update your plan, here is a guide to how often you should do it:

- Review/revise your annual plan quarterly.
- Review/revise your quarterly plan (within your annual plan) monthly.
- Review/revise your monthly plan weekly.
- Review/revise your weekly plan daily.

It's not enough just to create a plan — you have to *work* your plan.

As important as plans are, once you have created yours, spend the majority of your energy on the 'doing', not 'reviewing'.

Keep it achievable

A lot of people make the mistake of filling their daily, weekly or monthly plans with 101 actions when, deep down, they know that they could only ever achieve eight or ten of them. They believe that by writing everything down in the one plan, they will have a better chance of achieving their goals.

The problem with this approach is that ultimately it becomes demoralising and de-motivating, as you feel like you are only achieving 10 per cent of what you set out to do. A far smarter approach is to include in your plan only what you confidently believe you can achieve in the time available. Many of my clients who are achievement oriented have felt very uncomfortable with the idea of aiming only for what they know they can achieve, but one of the most important lessons for setting and achieving goals is that you set yourself up for success, not failure. By putting everything you can possibly imagine on your plan, all at once, you are just about guaranteeing your failure.

If you do feel you need a target that stretches you, add an extra task or two – but not 10! Choose activities you believe you will be able to achieve if everything else goes according to plan.

Remember, the more successful you feel, the more successful you will become, so it is a much better investment in your long-term success if your plan only contains things that you truly believe you can achieve.

Exercise

Take a moment to review the plans you created in the previous exercise (page 156). Are they achievable? Do you believe you will be able to achieve your goals within the time frames you have set?

There is nothing more important than setting yourself up for success, not failure – so take a moment to review your goals and make any adjustments necessary to ensure that you will achieve the *real* success and happiness you deserve.

THE WORDS YOU USE AND THE IMAGES YOU SEE

When it comes time to write up your plan, it's essential to consider carefully the words you use and the way you describe each step of your plan. You can apply what you have learnt about writing affirmations and the structures you used when writing your goals to the way you describe each step of your plan.

Instead of saying 'I will do x by a certain date,' say 'I have done x.' Use your plan not just as a blueprint or outline for what you are aiming to achieve, but also as an additional source of inspiration and motivation.

The richer and more emotive you can make your descriptions of each item in your plan, the more excited you will be about achieving that item. Even if the task is somewhat tedious or administrative, like completing the paperwork requirements before starting a new home-based business, if you are creative about the way you communicate your plan, you will feel much more enthusiastic about the things you need to do.

Even a positive statement like, 'I have completed the paperwork I need to start my new business' can be improved upon. How about following this statement with: 'I have cleared the path to my business success.' That feels much more exciting to me!

Because you are writing a plan, not just a list of affirmations, each of these statements needs to be followed by a completion or due date. For the more complex or time-consuming items, include a start date.

When you describe the objectives you are working to achieve in a way that calls a vivid image to mind, you will find that you are automatically visualising your future while you work at creating it. As you already know, visualisation is a powerful tool for creating the right subconscious foundations for your future.

If you are a visual or creative person you might even like to clip images from magazines or the Internet and attach them to a calendar to create a visual map of your plan.

However you choose to approach the creative part of planning, take the time to complete your plan in a way that supports your vision through affirmations, imagery and anything else that is generally inspiring to you. By doing this, you will find that completing items on this plan is not only easy, but also exciting as you watch your future unfold.

THE POWER OF THE PERFECT MONDAY

The most important day of the week is Monday. If you can get your Monday right, somehow the rest of the week just follows. I'm sure many of you have had the experience where at the beginning of the week things haven't gone according to plan and you have felt like giving up and starting again the following week...

Take the time to plan your Monday. Whatever you want from your week, focus on making it happen on Monday and it will be so much easier to keep up your good work for the rest of the week. Perhaps you want to exercise before work, communicate more assertively at work, eat three healthy balanced meals or be home from work early to spend time with your children. Whatever your goal, take extra care to make it happen on a Monday.

Give up Monday-itis forever and be eager to start the week right, knowing that when Monday works for you, you will find it so much easier to make the rest of the week work, too.

Exercise

Getting Monday right is one of the most motivational things you can do. Make a note of the things you would like to achieve each Monday to set yourself up for a week of success. You might like to include diet, exercise and 'me' time as well as professional goals such as specific meetings or reports that you need to complete. Again, make sure that the plan you have created for your perfect Monday is achievable.

When you are comfortable with your plan for a perfect Monday, write it down and put it in a place where you will see it regularly. It might be your fridge, your diary, your bathroom mirror, or all three.

Make sure you commit to achieving your goals each Monday – if you set yourself up for success at the beginning of the week, you will find that the rest of the week follows.

THE HARDER YOU PLAN, THE LUCKIER YOU GET

You've heard the expression, 'the harder you work, the luckier you get'. Well I have a small change to that: the better you plan, the more you will be able to seize all the luck coming your way.

Every day, life throws many, many opportunities our way, but most of us are so busy with our day-to-day existence that we never notice all of the exciting opportunities that turn up right on our doorstep. When we know where we want to be and we have taken the time to work out what we need to do to get there, things start to fall into place to help us along the way!

Some people call this fate, others call it serendipity, and some would say it is simply coincidence. You might believe that God is answering your prayers or that the infinite universe is delivering. Whatever the source of these opportunities, when you are clear about what you have to do to achieve your dreams, it is easier for you to see, accept and act on these generous gifts as they come into your life. The harder you plan, the luckier you will get.

Kyle's story

Kyle dreamt of becoming a celebrity chef. He had the personality and he knew he had the talent, but something was missing. He worked hard and the restaurant he worked in was well respected, but he just couldn't seem to get the break he needed to make it into the big time.

Although Kyle though he had a clear vision for his dream, he had never taken the time to create clear goals or build a plan that would take him to the future he so deeply wanted. He told me that he was worried that he just wasn't a lucky person. He could see his competitors gaining in profile and credibility. Some even had cooking programs on television and wrote columns for national magazines. Kyle couldn't understand why someone wasn't offering him the same opportunities.

After he created a plan that would help him achieve the recognition he knew he deserved, I asked him to reconsider the idea that he hadn't been lucky up until now. Some of the opportunities that had come his way were the chance to cater for a film premiere and for the birthday party of a celebrity. On each occasion, Kyle had turned the opportunity down because he couldn't see it as an important stepping-stone to achieving his vision. All he had seen were small profit margins and big headaches!

Now that he had a clear plan, he knew exactly what kind of opportunities he was looking for. Realising that he had, in fact, been very lucky up until that point, Kyle chose to believe that his luck would continue. There was simply no way he was going to miss the next golden opportunity to cross his path.

GET IN THE MOOD

Whenever you are preparing for a planning exercise, it's important to get into the right frame of mind. It may take you a while to create your plan, so it's also important to ensure you have allowed sufficient time and that you will be undisturbed for that time.

You might have a special space you sit in when you plan. I always like to work on my plans in my dining room, which has a sweeping view of Sydney's city and harbour. Such a stunning backdrop reminds me that the future is filled with infinite possibilities.

You might like to find a space that has a beautiful view, perhaps by the beach, out in the country or somewhere from which you can see the city lights.

If you are a more auditory person you might be inspired by certain styles of music. You might find a particular piece of music uplifting and inspiring in a way that makes working on your plan feel like pure pleasure.

Or you might like to fill a vase with fresh flowers or burn a scented candle, sit in a particular chair, wear a certain jumper or write with a particular pen.

Every person is different, so take the time to discover what makes planning a pleasure for you.

A BLUEPRINT FOR YOUR FUTURE

Whatever you have felt about planning up until this point — whether it is a fear that it would take the spontaneity out of your life, a history of creating unachievable plans, or spending too much time planning and not enough doing — it is time for a fresh approach.

I want you to view planning as an exciting activity, something you do to invest in your ideal future. Creating your plans shouldn't feel like a chore. After all, when you create a plan, what you are really doing is designing your future!

KEY LESSONS – BUILDING A DETAILED PLAN OF ACTION

1. Having a plan significantly increases your chances of getting to where you want to go – in the shortest possible time, with the least number of deviations.

2. A plan doesn't need to be any more complicated than a list of things you are going to do, and the dates by which you are going to do them.

3. Use a daily plan to help you achieve your weekly goals, a weekly plan for your monthly goals and a monthly plan for your annual goals.

4. Set yourself up for success, not failure, by creating a plan that is achievable. After all, it's not enough to create a plan, you have to be able to use it!

5. Use the rules of affirmations and goal-setting to create a plan that is exciting and inspiring – one that motivates you into action.

6. Monday is the most powerful day of the week, so give up Monday-itis and commit to the *power of the perfect Monday*.

7. The more you plan the luckier you will get. Following your plan will help you to see and seize all the luck in your life.

8. Create an environment that makes planning a pleasure for you – after all, a plan is a blueprint for your future!

CHAPTER 8
Managing your resources

Regardless of your vision for the future and your goals, it will probably take time, money, energy or a combination of all three to create a life you really love. 'I can't afford it', 'If only I had time' and 'Maybe some other day' are three of the most common excuses people use for not achieving what they truly want with their lives. Of course occasionally there are more complex reasons why you might find you are not living your best life.

Before you conclude that your situation is complex and unique, examine your inner dialogue closely to see if the obstacles in the way of your *real* success and happiness are a lack of time, money or energy. When you learn to manage your time, your money and your energy as if they were the most valuable resources you have, resources that are critical to your ability to achieve your goals, creating the life of your dreams will be easier than you have imagined.

FINDING AND MAKING TIME

'If only there were more hours in the day!' I don't know anyone who hasn't expressed that wish at some point in their life. The only way you can get more out of your day is to be smarter about what you do, and how you do it, during the day.

Time waits for no man or woman. It's an old saying, I know, but it is true. The sooner you realise that you can't out-run, out-wit or out-manoeuvre time, the better. With the simple acceptance that time is making the rules, not you, working with time, or 'managing time', will become much, much easier.

When you find yourself trying to fit a 15-minute task into a 5-minute window, a 1-hour task into a 30-minute window, and trying to squeeze something into a day that really requires a week, remind yourself that it's not a battle you can win. There will only ever be 60 seconds in a minute, 60 minutes in an hour and 24 hours in a day. Accept this and work with it – not against it.

Most people greatly underestimate the time it will take to get something done.

Most people greatly underestimate the time it will take to get something done; consequently, they never seem to have enough time to get through all the things they want to do.

When you estimate how long it will take you to do something, triple your initial estimation. If you think something is going to take 5 minutes, allow 15; if you think it will take an hour allow three; and if it has anything to do with fixing your computer, allow a whole day!

If you overestimate the time you think it will take to do something, not only will you feel much less stressed as you work on each task, if you finish what you were working on early, it will be like a gift of extra time!

Another common mistake people make is to think that the best way to get more out of time is to multi-task. In fact, the less time you have available, the more important it is to focus on one task and complete that, before moving onto the next one. After all, getting 10 things 10 per cent complete won't achieve 100 per cent of anything!

It's important to prioritise your tasks and achieve the most important things first. Often people find themselves becoming so bogged down in stuff, that they never get around to working on the things that would actually improve or change their life for the better.

It's not enough just to prioritise, you have to be prepared to stick to those priorities. Don't let procrastination get in your way. Focus on what's important and do it – first!

Focus on what's important and do it – first!

Exercise

Make a list of all the things you regularly need to get done during the week. You might want to include things you need to do for work, plus all the tasks and activities you need to complete in your personal life. Alternatively, you might like to complete this exercise twice, once for your working day and once for the rest of your time. When you feel you have completed your list, review it and see if you can think of other tasks you regularly need to get done, add them too.

Next to each task estimate the amount of time you think you will spend working on that task. Remember that we usually underestimate the time it takes to get something done by about one-third, so unless you know the exact amount of time it takes, triple your initial estimation.

Once you are sure you have captured everything you need to get done, allocate these tasks to a weekly timetable. You might like to create one using a spreadsheet, or take a sample page from your organiser. Place the tasks in the timetable and move them around until you have created an efficient and effective week.

If you find you have more tasks than you have time, look at which tasks can be done less frequently or delegated to other people. You might even find there are things you spend your time doing that don't need to be done at all!

When you have finished this exercise, you will have created your ideal week, one that includes everything you need to do, but allows time for each task to be done properly and in a stress-free way.

MAKING MONEY WORK FOR YOU

Do you currently work for your money? Wouldn't it be nice if your money was working for you! One of your goals might be to create more money, perhaps through a business or investment success. On the other hand, your goal might be to do something that requires additional money, like taking a world trip, a sabbatical, or moving to a bigger house. Regardless of the vision you have for your future, never having to worry about money, because you already have all you need, is an idea many people find very attractive.

The first step to making money work for you is to clarify your current financial position. Understand the reality of your financial position: how much you have in savings, how much you owe, your assets and your liabilities.

There is little point in having $5000 in the bank earning you 5 per cent interest, if you have $7500 in credit card debt costing you 10 per cent in interest. Although you might feel like you are getting ahead, keeping your money in savings rather than paying off your debts, in this case, would actually be costing you money.

The next step is to work out how much it costs you to live. Do you really know what you spend in a day, a week or a month? Do you know where your money goes? Are you making regular savings or are you just living from payday to payday? Until you familiarise yourself with your regular essential outgoings and how much you spend on non-essential items, you won't know how much money you need if you are to get ahead.

Once you know your financial position – both your big picture and the everyday costs of your lifestyle – you can create a budget based on your essential expenses, optional expenses and savings objectives. If you earn a different amount each month or are paid irregularly you will also need to put some money aside to cover your essential expenses in leaner months. If you budget properly you might even find you can allocate some of your income to a charity or non-profit organisation.

Creating and sticking to a budget, is like having a crystal ball. You will be able to see your future financial position. You will know when any debts are likely to be paid off and you will be able to see yourself getting ahead financially.

If it is going to cost money to achieve your vision for the future, then include a savings or investment plan specifically for these goals in your budget. If your goals require you to borrow money from a bank, having a clear understanding of your overall financial position and how much it costs to live your life will make it much easier to work out how much you can comfortably borrow.

Once your finances are under control and your savings level has increased, you will be able to consider making some investments. While credit card and other short-term debt, used to purchase things that depreciate or drop in value, is dead money, borrowing money to invest in things that will appreciate or increase in value can be a sensible investment strategy. Unless you are particularly financially savvy, talk to your financial advisor or accountant about the right investment strategy for you.

Worrying about money is a big waste of energy; your financial position is well within your control. With a little effort and long-term commitment, you can create a future in which you never have to worry about money again.

Worrying about money is a big waste of energy – your financial position is well within your control.

Caroline's story

Caroline, a successful management consultant, had two big financial goals. The first was to buy her own home, the second was to achieve financial freedom through a property investment portfolio. When I first met Caroline she was feeling disillusioned. Although she had a little money in her savings account, she hadn't saved enough for a deposit on a home. She felt especially frustrated paying rent, knowing that her money was going towards someone else's financial freedom and not her own!

Although she was well paid, she found it hard to manage her money. She found that some months she was able to put a lot into savings and other months she was dipping into it. She felt like she was constantly taking one step forward and two steps back.

I asked Caroline the same question I ask any client with a financial goal: 'How much does it cost to be you?' She wasn't sure of the answer, so I asked her to review her bank and credit card statements and make a note of all her outgoings during the month. The first step was for Caroline to add up this list and see how much she *really* spent each month. She was shocked – it was quite a bit more than she expected.

When she had completed her analysis I asked her to categorise each expense as either compulsory or non-compulsory. Her compulsory items included rent, electricity, basic groceries, credit card payment and similar items. Non-compulsory items included things like eating out at restaurants, going to the movies, going shopping and going away for weekends with her friends. I also

(continued)

asked her to determine how much she thought she would be able to save each month, with a bit of careful planning.

Armed with this information Caroline was able to *plan* her monthly spending. She used her budget to ensure that when payday arrived, she first put money aside for that month's compulsory expenses, then she transferred the budgeted amount of money into her savings account, and determined what non-essential items she would spend the surplus on, depending on her priorities that month.

Caroline found that following this system was a great help. She could manage her finances much more effectively and watch her savings steadily grow. In less than a year she had saved enough money for the deposit for her first property and was well on the way to creating her own financial freedom.

Exercise

If you don't already have a budget, now is the time to create one if you want to start making your money work for you. Start by making a list of everything you spend during a normal month. You might find it easiest to use a spreadsheet program such as Microsoft Excel. Include all your fixed outgoings, such as rent or mortgage, insurance and loan payments as well as variable expenses such as going to the supermarket, out to dinner or fuel and transport costs. The best way to make sure that your list is comprehensive is to go through your bank and credit card statements, making note of every withdrawal or debit on your account. Just to be sure, check this list against the previous month or two to see if there is anything you have missed. If some of your bills are quarterly, such as electricity, gas or water, include one-third of this amount in your monthly expenses list.

Once you have completed your list, add up all the items and subtract this total from the total amount of income you receive each month. If you earn a different amount each month use the average of three or six months earnings to get a more accurate picture. When you know what you *usually* spend and how much you *normally* have left over for savings or how much you overspend, you can start to create a budget.

Examine your list for any unnecessary items, overspending, or items you can cut back on. For example, it is easy to spend about $10 each day just buying coffee, soft drink and a snack. If you were to cut out this expense each year you would save more than $2500. Check your budget for similar items. Don't be so ruthless that your budget becomes unrealistic, you want to make sure that it is achievable and that you can stick to it over time.

Once you have a new budget for your expenses, determine how much of your surplus you are going to allocate to your savings account, to investments or put towards paying off your debts. Take the time to extrapolate this amount over a year and see how far ahead you will be in 12 short months!

INVEST MONEY TO BUY TIME — SPEND TIME TO MAKE MONEY

Many people find themselves in the position of having enough money, but not enough hours in the day, or having plenty of time on their hands but no money in their pockets. If you find yourself in a solid financial position but constantly time poor, evaluate your budget and see where you could find some money to put towards additional support to free up some of your time. The most obvious choice is additional home help to save you doing household chores, which would immediately provide you with more free time.

You might find you are spending your valuable time doing things you are not even good at, simply to save money, where you could get a specialist in who not only could save you time, but would probably get things done in well under half the time it currently takes you.

Look over your week and identify tasks you spend your time on that you don't enjoy doing and could comfortably afford to hire someone else to do for you. Even if you can't afford to outsource this activity all the time, you may be able to stretch to having some help, some of the time.

Don't allow yourself to fall into a 'poverty consciousness', where you don't want to give up any of your hard-earned cash to create a better quality of life for yourself. After all, nobody lies on their deathbed and says, 'I should have done more ironing,' or 'I wish I'd washed the car more often.'

If your financial position isn't strong and you have time on your hands, but you are unable to spend it enjoying yourself because your current finances don't afford you that luxury, then make good use of that time by making money.

You could earn money directly by taking a second job or working part-time. Or you could use your time to make money indirectly by learning a new skill, or studying part-time to build up your skills to help you earn more money in the long run.

MAINTAINING YOUR HEALTH AND WELLBEING

Whatever goals you are working towards, you need to be in good health so you can enjoy the future you are creating. It's easy to find yourself focusing on one part of your life only to neglect another, but you must learn to make your health and wellbeing a priority. Not only will you look and feel better, you will live longer. And if you are going to make the effort to create your dream life, I am sure that you want to be around to enjoy it!

Take a moment to think about how you are currently living your life. Do you treat your body as your temple? Do you eat the best quality food that you can afford, making sure that you give your body the fuel it needs to provide you with an abundance of energy?

Is your main liquid intake water? Do you drink over 2 litres a day and enjoy coffee, alcohol and soft drinks as an occasional indulgence, rather than an everyday staple?

If these ideals couldn't be further from the truth and you know you are eating on the run, snacking on junk and treating alcohol or coffee as a water substitute, then it's time to stop being your own worst enemy and start realising that the investment you make in your health is the best investment you will ever make. There are lots of different ways to get back on track. You might want to look at your current diet and eliminate one negative aspect each week until you are living a much healthier life. Alternatively, you can go on a full detox regime to kick-start your system and quickly get back into good habits.

Remember, the more dramatic your strategy, the more likely you will feel worse before you feel better, so think sensibly about what will work best for you in the long term.

You might want to visit a dietitian or naturopath who can devise an eating plan especially suited to your needs. If you are overweight, underweight, pregnant or have a history of ill-health, make sure you visit your doctor for a thorough medical evaluation before making any changes to your diet or exercise regime.

Whatever goals you are working towards, you need to be in good health so you can enjoy the future you are creating.

BUILD AN ENERGY RESERVE — GET ENOUGH SLEEP AND EXERCISE

It's going to take energy to achieve your goals and that means both physical and mental energy. You might feel too busy to exercise, but it's important to make it a priority. The less exercise you do, the less you feel like doing; the more you do, the more energy you have, not just for exercise, but for everything else in your life.

Exercise doesn't have to take place in a gym. It could be as simple as walking into work or getting off the bus or train a few stops early and walking the rest of the way. Invest in a pedometer and set yourself a challenge of walking 10 000 steps per day. If you make that a regular part of your day, you will soon see your energy levels rise.

It's important that you do exercise that gets your heart pumping (cardiovascular exercise) as well as strength training to build your muscle mass. The fitter you are and the greater your muscle mass, the more energy you will have.

It is easy to confuse mental fatigue and physical fatigue. After a long day at work, you might feel too tired to exercise, but it might actually be your brain that's tired, not your body. Regular exercise will help you to tell the difference and, as an added bonus, it will help you to clear your head and relax, mentally and physically too.

If you want to build an energy reserve, sleep is just as important as exercise. If you are not getting enough sleep, your body misses out on essential restoration and recovery time. Remember, sleep deprivation is a form of torture, so make sure you are not torturing yourself by getting less sleep than you need.

If you find the opposite, that you are actually oversleeping, you need to do more exercise. It sounds strange – why would you want to do more if you are feeling tired? The truth is that when you oversleep you can be left feeling tired and sluggish for the rest of the day, even though you have had more sleep than you need. To break this habit, set your alarm and get up and exercise.

One of the best things you can do for your energy levels is to create a routine where you go to bed at a regular time and get up at a regular time each day. If you combine this with regular exercise your energy levels will soar and you will build an energy reserve in no time.

Exercise

One of the easiest ways to get your health and wellbeing, sleep and exercise on track is to create a wellbeing diary. You might have heard of keeping a food diary when you are aiming to lose weight; a wellbeing diary is similar, except that it covers a broader subject area.

Rather than buying a fancy notebook you might find it easier to use a small spiral notebook that fits in your handbag or pocket. At the beginning of your diary make a note of your goals for your diet, nutrition, exercise and sleeping patterns. Using a fresh page for each day, make a note of:

- what you have eaten including snacks
- what time you got up
- what time you went to bed
- how many hours total sleep you had
- what exercise you have done

Some people find it useful to keep a journal over time, others find that they use it for a month or two while they create good habits to get back on track. I find a wellbeing journal useful if I feel off track. I am quickly able to address any bad habits if I write them down each day.

NURTURE YOUR SPIRIT

Your most important resource in creating your best life is *you*! It's important to take care of yourself, not just physically, but emotionally, too.

Whatever you are working on, it's crucial to take time out and just *be*. If you are focused on achieving something all the time you can too easily forget to stop and appreciate what you already have. It's a cliché, but life really is a journey, not a destination, so make sure you are taking the time to enjoy the ride.

No matter how busy your life is, it's vital to have 'me time'. You might be lucky enough to afford a health retreat for a big dose of 'me time', but precious moments to yourself can be achieved by activities like walking the dog, reading your favourite book or magazine, catching a movie or watching the sun go down.

It's also important to find time to relax, unwind your mind and process everything you have been learning and experiencing. I can't recommend highly enough the power of meditation to quieten the mind, and allow you to just *be*.

You might also want to try yoga, a simple ancient exercise system that uses concentration on the body to calm the mind. Many power yoga devotees don't realise that the original purpose of the *asanas*, or posture, in yoga, was to reach a place where one could be entirely still and calm in body and mind.

Aim to make time every day for at least 20 minutes of quiet and uninterrupted time. While you can achieve this through meditation, you can gain a great benefit from sitting under a tree and quietly eating your lunch, or getting up 20 minutes before the rest of your family, so that you can start your morning in peace. Whatever you choose it's important to remember that this 'me time' is not a luxury, it's a necessity.

Your most important resource in creating your best life is *you!*

Exercise

Look at the weekly plan you created in the exercise on page 156. If you haven't done so already, allocate 20 minutes of 'me time' each day. Ideally this would be a 20-minute block, but if you need to, you can break it down to two 10-minute blocks or four 5-minute blocks.

If you do need to break down your 'me time' into smaller chunks, make sure you don't let them disappear altogether. Aim to allocate 20 minutes of uninterrupted time to your weekly plan on at least two occasions — you will definitely feel the benefit.

FIND A BALANCE

With all of the things going on in your life — day-to-day activities, working on your goals, exercising regularly and spending time with family and friends — attempting to balance it all can easily become overwhelming. At times like this it's important to remember that it's not about being perfect, it's about being the best you can be.

There is no need to worry if you don't live every single day in perfect balance. Instead, focus on achieving *overall* balance in your life. If you aim to balance out the things that matter to you over the course of a week, or even a month, then ultimately you will still have achieved a balanced life.

Take time at the beginning of each month to look at your diary and think about how you will be spending the majority of your time. Then schedule the items you know are most likely to be missed when you are busy or under pressure. You might need to schedule your exercise sessions, a massage, or perhaps some quality time with your family or a 'date' with your significant other. Put these activities in your diary and treat them as seriously as you would any business meeting.

If you work towards creating balance over time, not only will you achieve it, you will feel less pressured and stressed than you would if you force yourself to attempt balance in every moment of every day.

CREATE A SUPPORT TEAM

As you work towards creating the life of your dreams, you don't need to rely solely on your internal resources. There will be a myriad of people you will be able to call on to support you.

Look around you at the people in your life. Who can you call on to be a part of your support team? Not everyone you know will fit the bill. Some people will be too busy, others too critical or judgmental, and some may simply be people with whom you don't have that level of connection, but within your circle you should be able to find two or three people you know you can count on to give you 100 per cent support along the way.

It's important to remember that you are not looking for people who can achieve your dream life for you! You're still going to be the one doing the work, but your support team will make it so much easier for you, giving you encouragement, support and generally cheering you on.

Depending on the type of goals you are working towards, you might also want to include some experts in your support team. Again, your experts won't be doing the work for you, but they will be on hand to provide you with the advice and the subject-specific expertise you need to make your goals a reality.

You might want to work with a professional coach who can support you across a variety of goals, or find a different expert for each of your goals. If you want to lose weight, then you might have a personal trainer or nutritionist in your support team, providing you with expert advice on what to eat and what type of exercise to do. If your goals involve your finances then you might want an accountant, financial advisor, property agent or stockbroker on your team. Business goals might need the support of a consultant, advisor or business coach. If you simply want to relax more, you might find a massage therapist or yoga teacher to be a valuable member of your support team.

There are also a wide range of support groups and networks that you can tap into for additional support in achieving your goals. From Weight Watchers® and women's networks to young entrepreneurs' groups, business groups, chambers of commerce and investor clubs, there is a network or support group for just about everything. Most are very affordable and hold events and seminars in which you can not only learn more about how to achieve your goal and be inspired by those who have gone before you, you will also meet like-minded people on a similar path who will share their experiences. You might even make some new friends!

Sam's story

Sam found running his business a rewarding but isolating experience. Although the business was going well, there were always things to worry about – staffing issues, strategic plans, short-term cash flow challenges and troublesome clients. He didn't feel it was appropriate to discuss the details of the financial operations with his staff and at the same time he didn't want to bore his wife with stress-filled tales of life at the office, or seem ungrateful by discussing his business issues with less successful friends. It seemed life was lonely at the top.

When I met Sam he was highly stressed and at risk of burning himself out. As much as he loved his work, he wasn't sure if he wanted to do it anymore. My first priority was to coach him in building a support network. I asked him to investigate networking groups to find out which ones might meet his needs. Sam chose to join a young business owners' group, which had been established specifically to support young independent business-owners. Through this group, Sam would meet men and women in a similar position to himself. He would have people to talk to who would understand *exactly* how he was feeling.

Next Sam needed to find a mentor, someone older and more experienced. He found his mentor, Mike, among his parents' friends. Mike had built several successful businesses over the

(continued)

years, but was now semi-retired. He was delighted to take on the role of supporting a younger man in business and quickly became a trusted ally for Sam, someone with whom he could discuss his business challenges and whose advice and wisdom he valued.

With his support team in place, Sam felt much of his recent stresses melting away. In no time he was back to his usual high energy levels and his business continued to go from strength to strength.

Exercise

Who would you choose for your support team? Write down the names of two or three people you know you can count on for unconditional support as you work towards your goals. If you don't feel you know who these people are just yet, don't worry, just keep your eye out for them. It might not be someone you are closest to, or someone you see often.

Next look over your goals and your vision for the future and see where you think you will need expert support. Make a note of the names of experts you tend to call on for support when you get to that stage of your plan. Again, if you don't know who these people are just yet, don't panic. Start asking your friends and family if there is someone they can recommend. Keep your eyes and ears open and your experts will appear in no time.

Then identify two or three support groups, networks or associations that will be of use to you while you work to achieve your goals. Alternatively, you might like to find a group of people who are working on a similar goal and create a support group or network of your own.

Make sure you are bringing all the people into your life you need to support you as you create the life of your dreams.

YOU HAVE EVERYTHING YOU NEED

You might not realise it yet, but everything you need to achieve your goal is well within your reach. Some things might be at your fingertips and finding others might require some effort and commitment on your behalf. If you manage your resources carefully and choose your support team wisely, you will soon have everything you need to achieve your goals.

KEY LESSONS — MANAGING YOUR RESOURCES

1. Work with time, not against it. Remember to overestimate the time it takes to get things done, work out what your priorities are and focus on doing one thing at a time. If you are able to get things done faster, it will be like receiving a gift of extra time.

2. Your financial future is well within your control. Don't just work for your money, make your money work for you.

3. Spend money to buy time by outsourcing things you can afford to pay others to do. If you have more time than cash, put that time to good use by doing things that will help you make more money.

4. The best investment you will ever make is in your health. Eat well, drink lots of water and remember that your occasional treats should be just that – occasional.

5. Make sure you're not torturing yourself with sleep deprivation. Keep your energy levels high by getting enough sleep and doing plenty of exercise.

6. Life is a journey, not a destination. Make sure you enjoy the ride by finding a little time to just *be* every day.

7. You don't need to be in balance every minute of every day to have a balanced life. Work at creating balance throughout your week or month.

8. There is no need to go it alone. Create a support team of experts to provide you with information, and friends and family to cheer you on.

Step 3

DO IT!

CHAPTER 9
Developing amazing self-discipline and staying power

At the beginning of this book, I explained that creating the life of your dreams is possible if you follow some simple steps. What I didn't say is that it is easy or instant — a big difference!

One of the most important things you can do if you want to have *real* success and happiness in your life is develop self-discipline and staying power. You really can have everything you want in life, but you must be willing to work for it. Sometimes it will be easy to follow the path you have chosen, but at other times it might not be. You will have to be focused and remind yourself why you have chosen your particular journey in the first place.

If you find it hard to be disciplined, don't worry — so do I! I'm not talking about waking up one day with discipline of steel, but instead developing the skills that build your discipline so that you can achieve all the staying power you need if you are to achieve your ultimate goal — the life of your dreams!

One of the most important things you can do if you want to have *real* success and happiness in your life is develop self-discipline and staying power.

FINDING IT HARD TO BE DISCIPLINED?

Your frame of mind can have a big impact on your ability to be disciplined. Do you have a limiting belief about yourself and your capacity to stick at something you have set out to do? Perhaps you have started things in the past that you haven't kept up with, or dropped out of a course or even a degree program? Maybe you have several half-knitted jumpers you never seem to get around to finishing off, or you can't seem to make yourself get to the gym regularly?

If there is anything in your past that you believe demonstrates you have a difficulty with discipline and staying power I want you to forget about it *right now!*

By focusing on past experiences in which you have disappointed yourself or others, you will only be reaffirming the limiting belief that you lack discipline or staying power.

The first thing you need to do is adopt a new mindset, one in which you are able to achieve any goal you set out to achieve. In your new mindset you recognise that achievements don't just fall out of the sky and acknowledge that you are the kind of person who is willing to work for what you want. You are the kind of person who enjoys the results of your efforts.

If you find it hard to stay on track, be that sticking to a new budget, keeping up with a course, maintaining a new fitness schedule or researching and writing your business plan, don't be angry with yourself. There is absolutely no point in beating yourself up because you feel like giving up or taking time off. Berating yourself won't achieve anything except lowering your sense of self-worth and eroding your belief in your ability to achieve your dreams.

Instead, I want you to go back to the notes you made about your vision for the future and read them – over and over! When you feel your staying power waning, rather than trying to rev up your discipline levels or giving yourself a harsh talking-to, focus your energies on the reason behind what you are doing. What is the vision that is driving you? What are the values you want your life to be in alignment with? What is your dream? And could you really risk letting the chance to achieve it pass you by?

By focusing on the future you are working to create instead of any difficulties or frustrations in the present, you will find your inspiration all over again. You will feel motivated to get there as fast as you can.

ARE YOUR GOALS THE RIGHT GOALS FOR YOU?

If you are really finding it difficult to be committed to your goals, and this is not just a bad day or a case of the blues but a serious commitment issue, then you need to go back and examine the goals you have set for yourself in the first place. When you look at the vision you have designed, ask yourself the question: 'Who is this all for?' If you are not sure of the answer then go back to your dreams and values and review the vision you have created. Make sure it is one that you are truly engaged with, one that excites and inspires you on the deepest level.

If you are not feeling that way about your vision then you need to ask yourself, 'Who am I trying to satisfy?' If you are honest with yourself and find that you are actually trying to impress others or fulfil the expectations of someone else, then nothing will help you to become more disciplined. In fact, your subconscious will actively work to undermine your progress if your goals are serving someone else's objectives for your life and not your own.

I call these 'coulda', 'shoulda', 'woulda' goals — goals based on things that you could do, or feel that you should be doing, or that you would do, if only you didn't have to work for them. 'Coulda', 'shoulda', 'woulda' goals are often created when you attach yourself to other people's expectations of your life — you are not being true to yourself. If your goals are not authentic, real and personal goals for you, then motivating yourself to do what you need to do to achieve them will be very difficult indeed.

Make sure that the goals you are working towards are not only meaningful to you, but that you believe in your heart of hearts that they are worth working for. Know that the dream life you are working to create is something you can not only achieve, but that you absolutely deserve.

DO YOU BELIEVE YOU CAN BE SUCCESSFUL?

Sometimes you can be your own worst enemy. The biggest obstacle getting between you and your motivation to achieve your goals could actually be your lack of belief that it will all be worthwhile. If you can't see how your current tasks fit into your bigger picture and how they are going to take you one step closer to your vision for the future, then you need to revisit your plan and see if they are really an essential element of your plan.

Or perhaps stopping you from feeling like the task at hand is worth it is that, deep down, you're not convinced that *you're* worth it — that *you* deserve to live your best life and that *you* have the power to create it.

If some limiting beliefs have crept back in, you might no longer be convinced that your goal is achievable or you may feel you are moving headlong into almost certain failure. If that is the case it is time to review what you have learnt about limiting beliefs and refresh your strategies for overcoming any lingering limiting thoughts you have or new ones you may have developed (see Chapter 3).

Watch out if you find yourself engaged in an inner dialogue that is similar to:

- It will never happen.
- I'll never be good enough.
- I don't know why I thought I could do this.
- I don't know why I bother.
- I just can't do it!

Replace these negative statements with strong positive affirmations. If you have grown tired of your old ones, re-word them and make them more dynamic. Concentrate on ensuring that they are positive, present tense and personal and start them with phrases like: I am, I have and I do.

Remind yourself that *it will happen*, because *you are good enough* and that you definitely *can do anything that you put your mind to*.

Don't be afraid to revisit the work you did in Chapter 3 on defeating your limiting beliefs. You will overcome some beliefs for life the first time you work on them, but others may rear their ugly heads at difficult or challenging times. Remember, reframe your thoughts with logic, reform your thoughts with affirmations and then move on. Don't let your inner critic get the better of the wonderful future you are creating for yourself.

SET YOURSELF UP FOR SUCCESS, NOT FAILURE

If you are finding it hard to achieve the staying power you need to reach your goals, take some time to look at the actual goals you have set yourself. Do you truly believe they are achievable?

Setting yourself unachievable goals is another major cause of de-motivation that can make sticking to your plan of action really tough. Even if you believed your goals were achievable when you set them, with the wisdom of hindsight would you still say that they genuinely are?

Perhaps you underestimated how long it would take to complete some of the tasks you set for yourself. Or, maybe you overestimated the amount of time you would have available to work towards your goals.

If you suffer from an over-achiever complex from time to time (see pages 129–30), you need to be especially mindful that you don't fall into the habit of setting yourself unachievable goals, and then giving up on them and feeling like you are a failure.

If you are the kind of person who wants to win, but is willing to walk away at the first sign that the prize might not be yours, now is the time to work on a new approach to the future, one where you commit to working towards your dreams, step by step, bit by bit, until they become your reality.

One of the most common mistakes people make when they begin to set goals is to become so excited and committed to their plan that they assume everyone and everything around them will feel the same way. They believe everything will go according to plan and sometimes it just doesn't!

Instead of letting what really amounts to a minor setback erode your commitment and staying power, go back to your goals and your plan of action and review them. Based on what you have learnt, is your plan still achievable? Were you as realistic as you thought you were being or would *naively ambitious* be a better description of your first plan?

If you discover that this is the case, don't be put off. Remember that your plan is a work in progress. It is not set in stone. You can't see into the future, so how can you possibly know how everything is going to turn out. Your plan is there to guide you, but if you need to make changes to it – do it!

There is no crime in amending or updating your plan. It's your plan and you can change it any time you like. Even if you decide that you have set yourself too much hard work and need to ease off a bit, no problem, it's your plan, you make the rules!

What does matter is that you change your plan consciously and knowingly. It is OK to revise your timelines and your expectations so that you can reinvigorate your commitment. The most important thing is that you don't use your initial unrealistic expectations as an excuse for giving up. Whatever you do, don't let your dreams just drift away.

Monique's story

The owner of a successful catering business, Monique's goal was to create a product line she could sell in gourmet delicatessens and supermarkets. When I met her she was feeling frustrated and de-motivated as she had set a goal of getting her product into the shops in the next six weeks and even without a detailed plan, she could see that at this point she wasn't going to achieve her goal.

One of the first things I discussed with Monique was the importance of setting yourself up for success, not failure. I challenged her on whether or not she really believed that six weeks was a realistic goal for the creation and distribution of a new product. She admitted it was unrealistically ambitious, but countered by saying that she wanted to be a high achiever. When I asked her how long she thought it took most businesses in the food and beverage industry to develop a new product and get it to market, she said 6 to 12 months and immediately acknowledged that a more appropriate goal for a *high achiever* might be to aim for six months.

(continued)

Once Monique set about creating a detailed plan for her products she could see exactly how unrealistic her initial goal had been. Rather than feeling discouraged by this discovery, she felt more motivated than ever, now that she could see exactly what she needed to do, and by when.

By following her plan, Monique was able to see on a week-by-week basis how much closer she was getting to her goal.

CREATE POSITIVE HABITS

One of the best ways to maintain your staying power is to set your discipline aside and focus on creating good habits. That's right, just forget about discipline altogether for a moment. Instead, I want you to think about all the things you could be doing to make sticking to your goals easier.

Anyone who has ever been on a diet will know that one of the essential first steps is to remove all sources of temptation from your cupboards and fridge and to replace them with healthy options. Suddenly you have a lot more staying power because you are not tempted to stray every time you walk past your kitchen. You can apply the same principle to your whole life. Remove yourself from temptation to stray and replace that temptation with new positive habits.

Discipline requires inner strength, will and determination. Habits, on the other hand, are something we have the ability to create in a relatively short time frame. Think about a bad habit you may have had in the past. How quickly did it take to develop from something you thought about to something you did automatically? It was probably only a couple of weeks.

We often only think of habits in terms of bad ones that we need to break, but we can use our habit-forming ability to our advantage. Habits don't just have to be for obvious things, like diet, exercise or budget goals; you can create good habits to support you in just about everything.

You might find you do need to be disciplined to create a new, positive habit, but it will only be for the first three or four weeks. By then you should find that you have developed a new, more useful way of operating that makes achieving your goals much easier.

Instead of constantly relying on discipline to keep you going, which can feel quite tough, invest your energy in creating habits that will soon become so automatic that you can save your discipline for life's real temptations!

One of the best ways to maintain your staying power is to set your discipline aside and focus on creating good habits.

Exercise

Look at the goals you are working to achieve and ask yourself which positive habits would support you in developing the staying power necessary to achieve your goals. Make a list of at least four new habits and make a commitment to develop one of these new habits each fortnight until you find that working towards your goals is something you do with ease.

THE IMPORTANCE OF MAKING GOOD CHOICES

Everything in life is a choice. It doesn't always feel like that, but it's true. You might be aware that you choose the clothes you will wear each morning, but you are also making other choices continually through your day.

You choose whether you should go to your meeting early, or try to squeeze one more task in; whether or not you want to exercise at the end of a long, hard day; and whether you want to meet your challenges head-on or take an easier road.

When you find it hard working on the things you know you need to do to achieve your goals, remind yourself that everything in life is a choice and that you are choosing to work towards creating the life of your dreams. Then make a conscious choice to do whatever it takes to get you one step closer to that vision.

A great way to identify times when you might not be making the best choices is when you say 'but'. 'But I didn't have time', 'but I was hungry', 'but so-and-so didn't do what I asked them to do'. I'm not saying these explanations will never apply, it's just that every time you say 'but' you are making an excuse – an excuse you most likely needed because you didn't consciously make a particular choice.

Everything in life is a choice.

Contrary to popular belief, things don't just *happen* in life. Every action you take has consequences, some more positive than others. If you had made a different choice you might not have needed your excuse.

Whatever goal you are working towards achieving, it's important that every choice you make supports the achievement of that goal. Not all your choices will be easy, but if you focus on the end result even the toughest of choices will be worth the effort.

Exercise

Take a moment to examine the level of choice you currently exercise in your life. Make a note in your journal of the things you do automatically that might not need to be done that way, or at all. Look at the times you are likely to use the word 'but' as an excuse for not achieving what you wanted to achieve.

For each 'but', make a note of the alternative choice that would have taken you closer to, not further from, your goal.

Make a commitment to live 'consciously'. Don't allow life to just *happen* to you. Make conscious choices about the goals you want to achieve and the things you need to do to make your dreams a reality.

HAVE A DEEP DESIRE

Getting to where you want to be in life does take effort. To make it easier for yourself, you need to know deep down that what you are working towards is something you *really want*. You have to have a deep desire to achieve your goals.

Instead of focusing on the effort you are going to make, focus on the outcomes you want to achieve. If you concentrate hard enough on where you are heading, what you have to do to get there won't feel so tough after all.

Focusing heavily on every single step you need to take to achieve your goal can make it difficult to motivate yourself. Instead, just focus on the step you are working on now. At the same time, keep the big picture in mind and remind yourself what you are ultimately working for. It might be tough keeping to a daily budget, but if you focus on an end goal – like becoming debt free or taking a sabbatical or the holiday of a lifetime – it will be much easier to maintain your staying power.

It is also essential that the goals you are setting yourself are attractive. They need to be meaningful and inspiring at the deepest level. Focus 100 per cent on what your goals mean to you. Perhaps your goal is to lose weight, but you are finding it hard to stay motivated. If you focus on something that is exciting and inspiring to you, like being able to run around and play with your children, your goal will immediately become a lot more meaningful and easier to achieve.

Likewise, if going back to university to study for your degree or postgraduate qualification is not exciting you anymore, focus on what you will be able to achieve with your higher education.

It's important to do whatever you need to do to stay focused on your vision for the future. If you are visual, you might want to create a vision board of images that inspire you to keep to your goals or you might want to use an image of what you are working towards as a screen saver on your computer.

If you're more auditory than visual, there might be certain songs that encourage and inspire you to make progress or work towards your goals. You might want to create a playlist for your iPod of music that sends your spirits soaring and inspires you to keep on going. Whenever I am running, if I start humming the theme from *Rocky*, I find it easier to run faster and keep going until I have reached my destination!

If you can keep your deepest desires at the front of your mind as you work towards your goals, the things you are doing won't feel like a chore, they'll feel like a pleasure.

KEEP YOURSELF ACCOUNTABLE

One of the best ways to stick to your goals is to be accountable for the work you are doing. This is why working with a personal trainer has become so popular. I once had a personal trainer I affectionately referred to as 'Running Man'. Running Man's job was simply to make me run. I found it so difficult to motivate myself to get up in the morning and run, but at the same time I knew from previous experience that if I worked on my running enough to build up my fitness, not only would I feel fantastic after each session, I would also enjoy the fabulous toning effect it had on my body.

One day a friend said to me, 'By using a trainer all you are doing is outsourcing your discipline.' 'Exactly,' I replied. I find it hard to get up early and go for a run, but I know that Running Man is going to ring my doorbell and will wake up the whole house unless I am at the door waiting for him. It really helps my motivation. And when I'm tired and beg to stop, he's not interested – which helps tremendously with my staying power!

There is nothing wrong with external support with your discipline and creating situations in which you have to be accountable for your progress. A personal trainer is just one example.

Another great example of an accountability structure is Weight Watchers®, which is both popular and highly successful in the results they help their members to achieve. At Weight Watchers® you are weighed and your progress is noted. There is no hiding whether you have been committed or not. At the same time, you are given great support from your team leader and other group members encourage you to keep up your good work and acknowledge the commitment you are making to your progress.

Working with a professional coach will definitely keep you accountable. Whether you are looking for personal, executive, business or career coaching, your coach will expect you to commit to certain actions at each coaching session and at the following session one of the things you will discuss is your progress against these actions.

Forming a support group, joining a network or finding a 'buddy' who is working on similar goals is another way to support yourself. You will have someone to be accountable to and report on your progress plus have a group of people with similar goals to support you and encourage you along the way.

Anthony's story

Anthony was a health and fitness trainer with an idea for a new group fitness program for middle-aged men. He needed coaching because he was having a lot of trouble with his own discipline and staying power. Although he had researched his idea quite thoroughly, he was finding it hard to take the next step – he would constantly start one task, only to find himself running in

(continued)

another direction and never getting back to achieving the task he had set.

What became apparent after spending some time talking with Anthony was his lack of belief in his ability to succeed. Intellectually he knew he could succeed. Logically he knew his idea was a good one, but somehow deep down he just couldn't make himself believe that he could do it.

Although he appeared confident, our coaching sessions uncovered a variety of limiting beliefs holding him back. I suggested that he work on his limiting beliefs using a series of powerful affirmations centring on his ability to succeed. Anthony needed to reform his thoughts and start thinking 'I have created my fitness program', 'I am successful', and 'I am living my dream life'. He also needed to learn how to create some positive habits that would support his staying power. Being a morning person, he agreed to allocate the first two working hours of each day to working through the tasks on his plan.

One of the main benefits Anthony gained from the coaching process was the accountability. At each coaching session he commited to completing certain tasks before the next session. Knowing that I would want to hear about his progress at the next session gave him the momentum he needed to complete his tasks.

With newfound self-belief and tasks he was accountable for completing, Anthony made great progress and his fitness program was up and running in no time.

AN ORDINARY LIFE WILL ALWAYS BE AN EASIER OPTION

Will achieving your goals be one long, hard slog? No. You will probably find that most of the time the knowledge that you are working towards your dream life will make tasks along the way a total pleasure.

On those occasions when striving for your goals does feel like hard work and your motivation is not as strong as it could be, remind yourself that an ordinary life will always be the easier option.

The fact that you have picked up this book means that an ordinary life is not what you are looking for. You want to live the best life you can, the life you have always dreamed of, and you are willing to work for it!

Getting to where you want to be in life does take effort.

KEY LESSONS – DEVELOPING AMAZING
SELF-DISCIPLINE AND STAYING POWER

1. Forget about goals you may have failed to achieve in the past. Instead adopt a mindset in which you are able to achieve anything you set out to do and then do it!

2. Don't fall into the trap of creating 'coulda', 'shoulda', 'woulda' goals in which you are trying to please everyone but yourself. Make sure that your goals are meaningful to *you*.

3. Overcome any limiting beliefs and learn to believe in yourself. You really can achieve anything you put your mind to.

4. Set yourself up for success, not failure, by making sure that the goals you have set yourself are genuinely achievable.

5. Focus on creating good habits that support you in achieving your goals. Save your discipline for life's real temptations.

6. Make good choices. Everything in life is a choice, so make conscious, positive choices that take you closer to, not further from, your goals.

7. Don't be overwhelmed by the detail. Focus on exactly what you need to be doing right now and keep your eyes on the bigger picture.

8. It's much easier to have discipline and staying power when you are accountable to someone for your progress. Create an accountability structure that works for you and the goals you are working to create.

CHAPTER 10
Facing your fears and calling on your strengths

Do you know what holds you back from achieving your potential? Have there been times in your life when a goal was in sight, but at the last minute you let it go or backed away? Chances are, whatever words you used to try to explain it, it was fear that was holding you back.

One of the most powerful questions I ask my clients is: 'What are you most afraid of?' Now I'm not talking about fears and phobias like spiders or aeroplanes, bridges or heights, or things that go bump in the night! The kinds of fears I mean are more subtle, much deeper fears – fears that sit at the bottom of your soul and eat away at your confidence, self-belief and self-esteem. If you don't invest the time and energy in overcoming your fears they will slowly begin to erode your sense of self-worth and ability to believe in yourself.

Fears can almost always be broken down into fear of failure and fear of success. Both fear of failure and fear of success are destructive in equal measures, so you need to be able to identify them and find a way of overcoming them.

Remember, it's OK to feel scared. In fact, sometimes feeling scared is a good thing. It shows that the things you want, and are committed to achieving, really matter to you. Fear itself doesn't have to hold you back. What does hold you back is the power you give those fears.

Exercise

Take a moment to think about the times in your life when you have allowed fear to hold you back. Perhaps there have been some significant events in which you did not achieve your potential because fear got in your way. Or perhaps there has been no one significant event, but lots of times when you weren't as courageous as you would have liked to have been.

Make a note in your journal about how you feel about these experiences now, what you have learnt from them and what you would do differently if you had the chance again.

ARE YOU AFRAID OF FAILURE?

Fear of failure has many guises, but it is most powerful in holding you back from achieving you potential. At first you might not even recognise that it is fear holding you back. You might think your concerns and worries are legitimate – and maybe they are, but if deep in your heart you feel you are not achieving your potential, a fear of failure is probably getting in your way.

Here are six common internal questions that signal a fear of failure. As you read through these questions, see if you recognise any of the fears described. Use the insights to assist you in examining your innermost thoughts and feelings and try to identify and overcome the fear stopping you from achieving your potential.

Remember, there is no such thing as failure – as long as you give your best you will always be a success.

1. What if I can't do it? What if I fail?

When you find yourself asking this question you are definitely experiencing failure-itis. Of course you don't know if you can do it if you've never done it before! When you find yourself questioning your abilities, it's important to remember that you will never know if you can do it if you don't try. And just like your mother used to tell you, 'If at first you don't succeed, try, try again.'

Tell yourself that it's OK if you don't get it right the first time. Remember, life is not about being perfect, it's about being the best you can be. Even if you have to give your best efforts several times over before you hit the mark!

There really is no such thing as failure, just lessons along the way to success. We have all heard the saying, 'It's better to try and fail than never to have tried at all.' It's true. Think of all the learning opportunities you would have missed out on in your life if you never tried anything new.

2. What if I'm not good enough?

Any fear of inadequacy is just a fear of failure in disguise. If you ask yourself this question you need to work on your confidence and self-belief. After all, you are good enough – simply because you are you! When you find yourself engaged in this sort of internal dialogue, you need to look at the limiting beliefs you may hold supporting the idea that you may be a failure before you even begin.

As with Question 1 above, you will never know if you are good enough if you don't try. To give yourself the best chance of succeeding you need to have self-belief – an inner sense that you are good enough and that you will succeed!

3. What if I let everyone down?

Another common fear of failure is that you won't just fail yourself, you will fail your loved ones and the people around you, too. If you work to achieve something you haven't achieved before, to set your life apart from the one you've been living, it is common to fear that if you don't succeed on your first attempt you will be disappointing all the people who believed in you and have been cheering you on.

Remember, the people you have chosen for your support team believe in you unconditionally and accept you for who you are. They are not expecting you to be perfect and will respect you for making an attempt.

As long as you give 100 per cent to everything you undertake, you don't let anyone down, regardless of your result. But if you give up halfway or never try at all, the one person you will be letting down is yourself.

4. What if I'm just kidding myself?

When you are working towards creating the life of your dreams, you are actually taking a risk. The risk isn't that you will succeed or fail. The real risk is that you will be changing your status quo, and once you start working towards your new life, you know there will be no going back.

You will no longer be able to be complacent about things that were once acceptable, and that is scary. You are afraid of failing and then being able to accept the life you used to live. You might be wondering if you are setting yourself up for failure or questioning if you have been realistic.

If you can see anyone else in the world doing what you have in mind or living the kind of life you desire, then it is realistic. Do you dream of being a bestselling author? Well, there are thousands of them, so of course it's possible. Want to retire at 45? Plenty of people do that too.

Remember, you create your own reality. You might not get there on the same timescale you had originally intended, but if you persevere, you will get there.

5. What if nobody likes me?

So many people crave acceptance. They seek external approval and validation from other people. If you find yourself engaged in an inner dialogue questioning whether people will like you, your fear is that you will 'fail' to be accepted.

One of the most powerful messages I have ever received was from a mentor when I was 18 years old. An incredibly successful businesswoman, she said to me, 'I don't worry if some people don't like me – in fact, I'm actually OK with it. After all, I don't like everybody I meet, so why would every person who meets me like me? As long as you like yourself, that's all that matters.' These were very powerful words for me as I set out on my adult life.

Remind yourself that it's OK if some people don't like you. That's their business and it actually has nothing to do with you at all. The good news is that if you are comfortable with who you are and you like yourself, then most people you meet will like you too!

6. What if people talk about me?

Another common manifestation of a fear of failure is the fear of being judged, the fear of being a failure in other people's eyes. You can't stop people from talking, but you can be mindful that the only source of genuine approval is from within. If you have that, you don't need anyone else's validation.

Be confident in your choices and the life you are creating for yourself. Hold your head high and don't let idle gossip hold you back from achieving your potential. The truth is, most people aren't thinking about you at all, they're too busy judging themselves and worrying what *you* think about them!

IS SUCCESS TOO SCARY FOR WORDS?

While most people are familiar with the concept of 'fear of failure', a lesser known, but equally destructive fear is the fear of success. At first you might ask yourself, how could I be afraid of success? Why would I be afraid of getting what I want?

The changes your success will bring might seem quite daunting, and subconsciously you might be questioning whether or not you will be able to manage the impact of your success. You might be concerned about becoming busier, receiving more attention and having increased responsibility or you might simply be worried that you won't like the future you are creating when you get there!

One of the most common manifestations of fear of success is self-sabotaging behaviour – when you literally become your own worst enemy and start doing things that actively move you away from your goal. Self-sabotaging behaviour might include getting drunk the night before an important job interview, binge eating when you are close to your weight-loss goal or becoming jealous and obsessive in a new relationship.

Addressing any fears you may have about success is just as important as learning to overcome your fear of failure. If you don't face your fears, you might subconsciously or even consciously undermine your progress and keep yourself at a *safe* distance from your goal.

A lesser known but equally destructive fear is the fear of success.

Examine the following six questions and see if you recognise any of them. Use the insights to coach yourself in overcoming your fears.

1. What if I can't cope with the attention?

One of the most common fears of success is that the progress you will be making will draw extra attention to you and not all of that attention will be welcome. Whether your goal is to achieve significant weight loss, create a successful business or write a bestselling novel, when you achieve your goal, people are going to notice!

For some people, their present circumstances allow them to prevent their star from shining. It's important to realise that in achieving your goals, not only are you being true to yourself and your dreams, you are also acting as an example to others who may not yet have found the courage they need to change their own life.

Be proud of the results of your effort. Acknowledge that it has taken courage, discipline and commitment to achieve your goals. If you focus your attention on the substance behind your achievement, you will quickly become more comfortable with yourself. As you begin to give yourself the acknowledgment you deserve, you will begin to accept the acknowledgment of others.

2. What if success makes me change?

Our social lives are often woven together with an intricate dynamic in which we all have roles to play. Perhaps in the past you were the fat but funny one, the frivolous party animal, or the serious career achiever. If you want to create a dream life for yourself, one of the things that may need to change is the role you previously played. You may become the slim and sincere one, the focused career guy or the stay-at-home mum.

Regardless of the role you play in life and how that may change as you work towards your goal, you are the one in control of the change. No one is forcing you to change. It is a choice you are making, and with that choice you can decide which elements of your persona you want to keep and which need to be updated.

One of the great discoveries you will make is that it is still the same you underneath. You are not becoming a different person. You are the same person, doing different things and making different choices. In fact, by living a life in alignment with your values you can only become more of your true self, not less.

3. What if I can't keep it up?

For some people, the biggest fear of success is the responsibility for maintaining their level of progress on a long-term basis. They fear they will be chained to their success.

When you are truly in control of your future, you will in fact be freer than ever. The longer you work towards your dream life, the easier it will become and over time, things that seemed so challenging in the beginning will feel like second nature to you. When you believe in yourself, you will find it easier to make choices that work towards your desired outcomes, not against them.

Remember, your goals are your own and you are free to change them or revise them at any time. It's important you succeed on your own terms and everything you are working towards supports you in achieving a life filled with *real* success and happiness.

Be honest with yourself. Don't give up on your goal just because you are afraid you won't be able to keep up with your success. Instead give your goals 100 per cent effort then consciously evaluate the satisfaction you receive from your progress along the way.

4. What if I don't like it when I get there?
Some people dream about achieving something for so long that when it's finally on their horizon, they become terrified. They are afraid they have been wrong all along and the goals they've been working for aren't the right ones at all.

It's important not to fear the future before it has happened. Do not doubt your ability to determine what is right for you. Remind yourself that nobody knows what is right for you better than you do. If you have taken the time to carefully construct your goals, which are the results of a clear vision and a strong understanding of your values, then it is extremely unlikely you won't enjoy the results of your efforts.

If on the rare chance you really aren't happy with your goals once you have achieved them, then that's OK too. Your mind is your own; at any point you can change it. Just because you have worked for something doesn't mean it has to be a permanent fixture of your life if you are no longer enjoying it.

It's your life and your choice. Simply adjust your sails and set forth for a new destination.

5. What if I am more successful than other people I know?

One of the reasons so many people feel afraid of success is that they fear they will upset the natural order of things in their life. Perhaps your current peer group is all of a certain income, education or socio-economic standard, but you know the goals you have set yourself will take you beyond what they have achieved, leaving you worried you will no longer fit in.

Whatever you do, don't let other people's position in life get in the way of your choice to create the life of your dreams. Unfortunately, there will always be a few people who resent your progress and success; fortunately they will be in the minority.

You are likely to maintain the most authentic of your existing relationships, at the same time as developing a new circle of friends and associates who will become your new peer group. If you can maintain your most genuine friendships while continuing to make new friends who share your interests, values and ideals, your life will be rich indeed!

6. What if people stop liking me?

As was the case with fear of failure, the thought of newfound success can make you feel vulnerable in your need for acceptance or approval from others. Remember that the most valuable people in your life are those who love and accept you unconditionally. These people are happy for you and excited about the changes you are making in your life. There may be people in your life that preferred the old you – not because of any negativity about your new direction, but because in changing your life you highlight the changes they wish they were making but have not yet found the courage to do.

Everyone is entitled to make their own choices in life and if people don't like the choices you are making, that's their problem, not yours. If they can't be happy for you, you may need to question your desire to maintain this friendship.

Exercise

When you are excited about the goals you are working towards, it can be quite a shock to find yourself sidelined by either a fear of failure or a fear of success. Complete the following question in your journal:

Succeeding at my goal means that I...

Keep answering this question until you have uncovered everything that success means to you. Make a point not to edit your responses or focus only on the positive. You want to identify *all* the different feelings you have about success so you can begin to address them one by one.

When you have completed this, repeat the exercise for this question:

Failing to achieve my goal means that I...

Again, keep answering this question until you have uncovered all the feelings you have about failing to achieve your goal. Once you have discovered *all* the feelings you have about failure, even those that may be conflicting or confusing, you can begin to address them.

ACKNOWLEDGE YOUR FEARS BUT NEVER GIVE IN TO THEM

One of the most powerful things you can do to overcome your fears is acknowledge them and then move on. Susan Jeffers made famous the phrase, 'Feel the fear and do it anyway', with her book of the same title*. Learning how to acknowledge your fears without giving in to them is one of the most important skills you can learn.

Your fears, like all of your other feelings, are yours. You are 100 per cent entitled to them and you should never feel as though you have to apologise for them. What is important, however, is to be mindful of how much power you give your fears – just because you are afraid of something, it doesn't mean you can't do it!

Instead, acknowledge your fear, accept that while it might not be particularly pleasant, it is how you feel, then carry on regardless.

Sometimes an acknowledgment is all you need to disempower your fear entirely. If you deny the fear or try to overcome it without first accepting that you feel it, you waste an inordinate amount of energy trying to conquer it, which simply might not be necessary.

Next time you find yourself experiencing any fears, examine them, accept them and then carry on regardless. It is one of the most empowering things you can do. Each time you do it, your self-confidence will increase dramatically!

---

* *Feel the Fear and Do It Anyway*, Susan Jeffers, 1987, Century.

Worst-case scenario

One of the most useful things you can do to manage your fear is consider the worst-case scenario. What is it, and would you survive? It's extremely rare that the worst-case scenario assessment identifies a situation you simply could not live with, or would never recover from.

When you find yourself afraid of failing or intimidated by the idea of success, ask yourself, what is the worst thing that could happen here? Keep asking yourself this question until you have reached the bottom of the idea pond and look at the outcome.

So often people find that the result of their worst-case assessment is actually something they could accept. They might not have ever chosen that outcome, but should it occur, they know that after a period of adjustment they would survive.

Exercise

Think about a fear you are experiencing. Ask yourself:

If my fear were to be true, what would be the worst thing that could happen?

After each answer, ask yourself the question again. Keep repeating this process until you are sure that the worst-case scenario is something, however unpleasant, you know you would be able to cope with.

Will's story

By the time he was 35, Will was the owner of a successful chain of juice bars and was considered somewhat of a wunderkind by his peers. He came to coaching by accident. We had met through an acquaintance, and my work piqued his interest. I suggested that if he wanted to find out more about coaching, he could make an appointment to come and see me.

The first thing Will told me during our initial meeting was that everything was great in his life – there really wasn't anything he could think of that he needed to work on. So I asked him if anything worried him or kept him awake at night. He told me he was worried if he was happy. He acknowledged that although he was highly successful, he wasn't having fun anymore. With each success his reputation had grown, as had the pressure to repeat it, and he was concerned he was beginning to burn out.

Will had fallen victim to his own image of success. He was trapped in a cycle of worrying what people thought and then resenting that their opinion mattered to him. He had begun to fear doing anything that could be perceived as failure.

I asked him to think of three things he would do if failure were not an issue. They didn't have to be work related, they could be about anything. He said he would employ a general manager to free up some of his time, learn to play the guitar, and get his private pilot's licence.

Will soon realised that the only thing stopping him from making these changes was fear, and he wasn't about to let this get in his way!

DO THE THING THAT SCARES YOU MOST

It's important not to view fear as a negative feeling. It can be an illustrative feeling. It allows you to see how you feel about something on many different levels – and gaining a better understanding of yourself is never a bad thing.

I have felt terrified many times in my career; afraid I would fail, that I wouldn't be good at what I had set out to do – or that I had bitten off more than I could chew! I never saw this fear as a bad thing. In fact, I even had a name for it. I called it *scary-good*. *Scary-good* is the feeling I get when I know something is very important to me and succeeding is really going to matter in my life.

I found a way to feel comfortable with these fears. I saw them as a good sign that I had taken on a new challenge and wasn't being complacent in my life. I also found this *scary-good* feeling to be highly informative. It enabled me to quickly separate experiences that mattered from those that weren't important. I became so comfortable with this feeling of being terrified for the right reason – if I didn't feel it when I started a new assignment or role, I knew I hadn't chosen a big enough challenge!

Learn to embrace all your feelings, not just those that leave you feeling warm and fuzzy. Make sure you take the time to acknowledge your 'negative' feelings – it's important for your personal growth and development.

It's important not to view fear as a negative feeling.

THREE SIMPLE STEPS TO MANAGING YOUR FEARS

Just because you are experiencing fear, it doesn't have to get in your way. Follow this simple three-step strategy for managing your fears:

Step 1 Reframe your thoughts with logic and objectivity

You will remember the art of reframing from Chapter 3. To recap, reframing is about giving yourself a stern talking-to. You might like to use the worst-case scenario analysis. Another favourite of mine is the statistical likelihood question: What is the statistical likelihood that everyone you know will judge you if you don't succeed at the first chance? Five or ten per cent of the people you know might judge you, and if you move in a particularly small-minded circle, maybe even 40 per cent, but the likelihood that every single person you know will be passing judgment is really so slim that it is hardly worth thinking about!

If, when you ask yourself this question, you come up with a response that has quite a high probability, then you need to work on addressing the scenario at hand. If there is a high likelihood your fear will be realised, mitigate that fear with actions. Don't give up on your goals to prevent the fear from becoming a reality.

Step 2 Reform your fears with powerful affirmations

I am a huge fan of affirmations. They are simple and efficient and they work. The fastest way to overcome a fear is to reform your thoughts so that the fear is simply no longer a part of your reality.

Examine the situation causing you to experience fear. Identify the source of the fear – success, failure or something more obscure. Then create a simple statement or phrase that turns your fear on its head. Don't forget to make sure your affirmation is personal, present tense and positive. You want to create a strong new message to reprogram that negative thought in your brain.

Think of a CD that is stuck on repeat playing the same negative fear or worry. Using affirmations is like taking out the disc and putting in a new one. You will still want to play it over and over, but this time you will be giving yourself confidence-boosting messages, not self-esteem-eroding fears.

Step 3 Take action

The most important step in overcoming your fears is taking action, regardless of how you are feeling. Many people mistakenly believe that if you are afraid of something, you can't do it. Of course that's nonsense. Even if you are frozen with fear there is still nothing physically stopping you from working towards your goals.

If you are feeling particularly courageous, you might want to take a big step and do precisely the thing that scares you the most. On the other hand, you might be feeling so much trepidation that you prefer just to take baby steps towards your goal.

Whichever approach you choose, taking action will have two main benefits. By working through your fear, you will reduce the power it has in your life. You will send your subconscious a clear message that nothing gets in your way!

The other important benefit of taking action is that *you will have taken action* – you will be a significant step closer to your goal and the life of your dreams will once again be within reach.

Kelly's story

When I met Kelly, she was a struggling author. She wasn't struggling in the financial sense – she had a day job as a journalist. Her struggle was that she simply couldn't make any progress on her book. She believed working with a coach would provide her with the structure and accountability she needed to make consistent progress on her book and turn it into a bestseller.

After talking to Kelly about her vision for the future as a successful author, it became apparent that a disempowering fear of both failure and success was getting in her way, not lack of discipline. Every time she sat down at her keyboard she felt paralysed and unable to write.

When I asked Kelly what she was afraid of she immediately answered that she was worried her book wasn't going to be good enough. I asked her to think a little more about her fears, and she added that she was worried she would feel a failure in front of her colleagues at the newspaper if it wasn't good enough, and if it was good, she might alienate her colleagues who were dreaming of writing a book but hadn't done anything about it. She also felt that if her book wasn't a success it might affect her general credibility as a writer, and if it was a success she would have to overcome her shyness and give public readings and interviews to the press.

When Kelly got all this off her chest, she immediately felt relieved. It hadn't occurred to this strong and successful career woman that her fears were getting in her way. At last she had an explanation for the difficulty she was experiencing in starting

(continued)

her work. Once she had identified her fears, Kelly was able to reframe her thoughts and reform her thinking. She examined her fears and replaced them with logical and objective thoughts about her current success as a writer and she created powerful affirmations that filled her with a deep sense of belief in her writing project.

Most importantly, Kelly took action. She set a regular time each week to sit down and write. Regardless of how she was feeling or what she thought about the words she was writing, she worked diligently and, before she knew it, her book was finished.

PROTECT YOUR FUTURE

When you are feeling overwhelmed by fear, it's important that the only actions you take are those that bring you closer to your goal. Your fears can cloud your judgment or influence your ideas of what you do and don't want in your life. When you are feeling afraid, it becomes easy to say to yourself, 'Maybe I never wanted that goal after all.' Many people miss out on their dreams because when the going got tough and they were filled with fear, they decided their dreams weren't worth pursuing after all.

Do not make any decisions that affect your future when you are in the depths of fear. Keep moving in the direction of your goals and wait until your fear has subsided before you re-evaluate the future you are creating for yourself.

GET PRACTICAL SUPPORT WHEN YOU NEED IT

Sometimes you actually need outside help to overcome your fears — try as you might, you just can't seem to overcome them. You might want to call on an expert for support. Perhaps you simply can't see a way around your fear. If you are afraid you won't be able to create a future that includes financial freedom you might want to call upon an expert such as an accountant or financial advisor to support you. Similarly, if your fear is about how you will manage your success, you could find a mentor who will give you the opportunity to learn directly from their experience and how they have managed the challenges of becoming more successful. Occasionally you might find your fears are so deep-rooted that you are unable to overcome them without the support of a trained professional and you might need to see a therapist or counsellor.

Never be ashamed to seek whatever kind of support you need to create your ideal future, even if it is psychological or emotional support. A brave person is one who is willing to do whatever they can to move on from their fears to a better life.

CALL ON YOUR STRENGTHS

One of the exercises you completed in Chapter 6 was to identify your strengths. Well, now it is time to call on them!

Everyone has a set of positive qualities that make us all unique individuals. When you find yourself experiencing fear of failure, success or a combination of the two, remind yourself that you actually have a lot going for you.

Your fears can leave you with a sense of inertia. You can feel as if you are trapped in your fears and unable to move forward towards your goal. Recognising your strengths can help to break this spell. If you spend some time thinking about all the things that are fabulous about you, you will feel re-inspired and motivated.

When you remember what *your* strengths are, you will know precisely why you *do* have the ability to achieve your goals. You will know that a risk of failure can't hold you back and that whatever challenges success brings, you will be able to take them in your stride.

Everyone has a set of positive qualities that makes us a unique individual.

LIVING YOUR BEST LIFE TAKES COURAGE

Never forget that it takes courage to create the life of your dreams. It will always be easier to choose a complacent life, never stepping out of your comfort zone or challenging yourself in any way. But is that what you want?

When you feel fear getting in your way, remind yourself that you are working to create a life filled with *real* success and happiness – not a life that is nice, fine or just OK. Take a deep breath and move through your fears. If you give 100 per cent effort to everything you do, the life of your dreams will be yours.

KEY LESSONS – FACING YOUR FEARS AND CALLING ON YOUR STRENGTHS

1. There is no such thing as failure. As long as you put in your best efforts, you will always be a success.

2. Success can be scary – it's inevitable that when you achieve your goals, some things in your life will change. Accept those changes and embrace the future you are creating.

3. One of the most empowering things you can do is acknowledge your fears and then carry on regardless.

4. Sometimes being afraid is a good sign – it lets you know that what you are about to do really matters to you. Embrace this as a positive feeling and do what scares you most.

5. Never let your fears get in your way. Remember this simple three-step strategy for managing your fears:

    Step 1 Reframe your thoughts with logic and objectivity.
    Step 2 Reform your thinking with powerful affirmations.
    Step 3 Take action.

6. Avoid making decisions from a place of fear. You will always make a better decision when you are feeling strong, confident and positive about your future.

7. Don't be afraid to seek practical support in managing your fears. Remember, asking for support is a sign of strength, not weakness.

8. You already have so many things going for you. Whenever you feel fear getting in your way, think of your strengths and call them into action!

CHAPTER 11
Working through the tough times

Just because you are committed to creating a life you love, it doesn't mean you will never have another bad day or nothing will ever get in the way of your dream life. While it's true that you will be so in control of your future that bad days will seem few and far between, I'd be lying if I said that everything will be perfect from this point on.

Real success is not about never having a bad day. What is important is how fast you can turn that bad day around, how quickly you can form a strategy to overcome any obstacles that may appear on your path and how fast you can recover from a disappointment or blow to your confidence.

The better you become at mastering the key lessons in this book, the faster you will become at mastering the turnaround from someone who is feeling disappointed or defeated to someone who is confident and in control of their destiny.

People often say to me, 'You must never feel de-motivated, you're an expert on motivation. You show people how to build their confidence, you must never have a day when your confidence is low.' The list goes on. Of course I have a bad day here and there, after all, I'm human not superhuman! The real difference is the speed at which I am able to turn my day around and the agility with which I can overcome obstacles and get back on track to my goals.

Everyone has tough times. Experiencing challenges and difficulties is not a reflection of character; how you manage and move through these times is.

OVERCOMING INTERNAL OBSTACLES

Sometimes the biggest obstacles in our way are our internal obstacles. These are barriers we alone are responsible for placing in the path of our *real* success and happiness. We create internal obstacles when we succumb to fear, self-doubt and limiting beliefs.

One of the best ways to identify an internal barrier to success is to pay attention to the times you find yourself saying, 'yeah but', 'but what if' or something similar. There really are no 'buts' on the path to success, just things you can work with and things you need to work around.

Don't let your 'buts' get in the way of your future. Take the time to examine your inner dialogue and observe the limiting beliefs, self-doubt and fears that have begun to take hold, and then use the tools and methods you have learnt about overcoming your limiting beliefs (Chapter 3), building unshakeable self-confidence (Chapter 6) and facing your fears (Chapter 10).

Reframe your thoughts, reform your thinking, acknowledge your fears or doubts, remind yourself that you can achieve anything you set out to do, and then carry on regardless!

ARE THINGS GETTING IN YOUR WAY?

As you work towards achieving the life of your dreams some setbacks will be beyond your control. Sometimes life does throw obstacles in your way. Fortunately, there are only two types of external obstacles; obstacles that are within your control and obstacles that are beyond your control.

If something is within your control, then look at what you have learnt about planning (Chapter 7) and managing your resources (Chapter 8) and make changes that will help you work around or resolve the issue sooner rather than later. You might need to adjust the timescale you were originally working towards, or add some additional steps in your plan. Or maybe you have discovered that achieving your goal is going to take more money or energy than you had initially realised, so you will need to build up your reserves in these areas.

If the situation currently holding you back is truly beyond your control, then you need to learn to accept it. Achieving a state of acceptance might be much easier said than done, but whingeing and wailing about things that are beyond your control is a waste of time and energy.

An obstacle in your path is not a reason to give up. While you might have to accept the current circumstances for what they are, never use this as an excuse to stop doing your utmost to create a life you love.

Don't make the mistake of believing this stumbling block is a 'sign' that you have been unrealistic or that you are foolish to try to create the life of your dreams – it's not! Everyone deserves to have real success and happiness in their life.

Use the disappointment you feel at this setback to re-confirm how much the goals you are working towards really do matter in your life. Use it to reignite your desire for your very best life.

> **As you work towards achieving the life of your dreams some setbacks will be beyond your control.**

IS YOUR OBSTACLE AN INTELLECTUAL ILLUSION?

Sometimes what is getting in the way of your success might seem like a real obstacle and it is, but at the same time it isn't. I'm not talking about an optical illusion; I am talking about intellectual illusions.

Intellectual illusions are obstacles you create when you fall into the trap of over-complicating things, of making things appear more difficult than they might really be, and of searching so hard to find the obstacles in a situation that you are able to see them even if they are not really there.

You might be telling yourself that you are just covering all the bases or thinking through the risks and issues, but what you are really doing is creating excuses in advance! Self-created obstacles or intellectual illusions are usually the result of a fear. Creating an obstacle allows you to avoid the risk of seeing your plan fail.

Exercise

What are the obstacles to your plan? What might affect the way you are able to go about creating your vision? Make a list of everything you can think of that could get in the way of your dreams. Don't worry about being negative, just get all your worries and concerns onto paper.

When you have captured everything you can think of, make a note next to each item as to whether it is an internal obstacle, an external obstacle that is within your control, an external obstacle that is beyond your control, or not really an obstacle at all.

Once you have categorised each item, review your list. This time, make a note of what you can do to overcome each internal obstacle. It might be to create an affirmation, to do some reframing of your thoughts, to work on your confidence or to create some new habits that will support your staying power.

For each item categorised as external but within your control, create a mini plan of action. What can you do to work with or around this obstacle?

Finally, for all the items you have categorised as external but beyond your control, I want you to make a decision that, should these obstacles arise, you will accept them. You won't moan or whine, but instead you will go back to your drawing board, reignite your passion and find a different way to reach your goal.

Self-created obstacles keep you in a safe place, one where you can't fail because you are not actually moving any closer to your goal.

If you feel you are creating obstacles in your path, ask yourself, What am I afraid of? It's most likely you will be experiencing fear of failure, fear of success or fear of the rejection that might occur as a result of your success or failure.

Use the tools you learnt in Chapter 10 to overcome your fears. Reframe your thoughts, reform your thinking and take action. You will soon discover that the obstacle you have imagined is not really an obstacle at all.

Tom's story

When Tom's wife passed away from cancer, he decided to establish a foundation in her name to raise funds for the hospital ward in which she had spent most of her time. He had a vision of buying comfortable sofas, *real* overnight beds instead of those wiry camp beds and maybe even a home cinema set-up — things that would make loved ones feel more physically comfortable during such an emotionally difficult time.

Tom was already familiar with goal-setting and started planning the foundation. Then he hit a stumbling block. To establish a foundation, there were a lot of legal and tax requirements. He was at a loss: not only did it seem like there were a million forms to fill in, but there were different requirements for different types of foundations. Having listened to his complaints that he wasn't making any progress, Tom's sister suggested that he try working with a coach.

(continued)

After discussing the progress he had already made on the foundation, his plans for fundraising and his ideas on the donations he wanted to make to the ward, I asked him if there was anything else getting in the way of the foundation. He was silent for a moment, then confessed that deep down he was afraid that he just couldn't do it, and that his attempt to make a difference would fail.

I admired Tom's courage in being so honest. Then I suggested that perhaps some of the headache over the tax and legal structures was an intellectual obstacle he had created to protect himself from failure. We spent the next few coaching sessions working on Tom's confidence and self-belief, which had taken a blow during the grieving process, until he truly believed that he could make this foundation a success.

Once he had overcome his intellectual obstacles, he realised the tax and legal issues had never been real obstacles and he was able to resolve them with a quick discussion with his accountant.

LEARN TO ASK FOR HELP

When things seem difficult, overwhelming or downright awful, it's important to seek the support you need to get back on track.

Just because you are working on creating a vision for your future, you don't have to go it alone. Look at your support team (see Chapter 8) and ask yourself if there are any other roles you should be looking to fill on your team.

The best way to resolve or work around your obstacle might be to bring in technical support – someone who can help you unravel the facts of the situation, find answers to complex problems or help you with the details or logistical aspects of your plans. At other times the support you need might be purely emotional. You might just need a bit of extra TLC from someone who is able to give you unconditional encouragement and support. Someone to whom you can say, I really don't feel great about this right now. Someone who will give you a leg up so that you can get back in that saddle!

You have your support team, but you do still have to ask for support. People aren't mind readers and we can all do a very good job of acting like things are OK, when quite frankly, they're not!

Practise asking for emotional support when you need it. Learn how to say, 'I'm having a difficult time at the moment and I would love your support.' Follow your request with how best the person can support you. Say something like, 'the best way you can support me at this time is…' Sometimes you might be looking for someone to listen, other times you might need someone to help you brainstorm a way forward. At times you might not want to talk about it at all, but will simply appreciate being in the company of someone who cares.

Occasionally you might need a more specialised type of emotional support. The tough times you are going through might require the support of a counsellor or psychologist if you are to make your way through them. Never be afraid to ask for expert help if you feel that is what you need. Asking for help is a sign of strength, not weakness. Have courage and seek whatever support you need to get you back on track and closer to achieving your goals.

> **Asking for help is a sign of strength, not weakness.**

IT'S TIME TO THROW A 'PITY PARTY'!

With all this discussion of being positive, overcoming your fears and managing your self-talk, you could easily believe you are never allowed to have an off day, a day when things are not going your way and you feel a bit down or that things are harder than they need to be.

Sometimes you actually need to take a little time out to lick your wounds and recover from the blow dealt by your disappointment. Feeling a little sorry for yourself isn't going to undo all of your hard work – as long as you don't let the feeling linger.

If you need to indulge your feelings, I recommend that you first decide how long you are going to allow yourself to feel blue, and stick to it. You might say: from 5 pm to 6 pm this evening I am going to sulk about this disappointment and then I'm going to get back to reviewing my plan and working out what I need to do differently.

Sometimes you might need a whole day. I call this a 'doona day' – where you just want to lie in bed and pull the covers over your head. And you know if you need to do this, it's OK. Again, it is important to decide how long you are going to spend licking your wounds. This will protect you from falling into the bad habit of letting this state of mind linger.

If you need to go to bed for the day and lick your wounds, do it. Having a mental health day or a day of recovery is a much better investment of your time than moping around feeling sorry for yourself for weeks on end because you never took the time to get over your setback properly.

Exercise

Take a moment to think of all the things that cheer you up when you are feeling blue. You might include things you like doing, such as going to the movies or listening to a live band, going to a park or walking on the beach. Maybe your favourite pastime when you're feeling down is to curl up on the sofa with a good book or golden oldie on DVD.

Make a list in your journal of all the things that are guaranteed to make you feel even a little bit better. By making this list now, when you do need to take time out to lick your wounds, you will know exactly what to do to make yourself feel better.

LOOK FOR THE LESSON

One of the most powerful things you can do when you are going through tough times or obstacles appear on your path is to look for the lesson. Everything we experience in life is an opportunity to learn — about ourselves, about other people, our ideas, values and beliefs. Sometimes it's just a chance to learn more about how things work in our business, workplace or relationships.

It isn't always possible to discover what the lesson is in the immediacy of the moment, but if you keep an eye out for the chance to learn something and remember that every experience presents an opportunity to learn, then tough times won't feel so worthless.

If you can look at everything you do in life as a chance to learn something new, then you will find it much easier to see the positive in every outcome. Even when things don't go according to plan or you find obstacles in your path, you will be able to see the point of every experience and the lesson within every disappointment.

Exercise

No matter how difficult things might be, there is always something to learn. Often we aren't able to identify the lesson at the time — it's only with hindsight that we can appreciate everything we have learnt.

Take the time to look back over your life and identify three difficult times or experiences. Even if you didn't realise it at the time, you learnt something from each of those experiences. Make a note in your journal of what you feel you learnt and how your life has benefited from that wisdom.

THE TIMING DIFFERENCE BETWEEN EFFORT AND REWARD

When things haven't gone your way, it's easy to fall into the trap of defining your situation as a 'failure'. But, really, there is no such thing as failure. As long as you're committed to what you're doing and confident that you've given it your best shot, you can never fail.

Some things in life are achieved the first time around; others take a little more time and a lot more practice. If you don't succeed the first time you try to achieve something, you certainly haven't failed. You have taken another step on the road to your goal and regardless of how it feels at that moment, based on all you have learnt, you will still be one step closer than you were when you started out.

Even though it's important to strive for success and focus on a positive outcome, it's also important to recognise that if you're not successful every single time you work on something, you haven't failed. Your plan might need tweaking, the goal might not have been achievable, the stars might not have been aligned, but you haven't failed!

Some things in life are achieved the first time around; others take a little more time and a lot more practice.

Success isn't always instant; you will inevitably experience a timing difference between all the effort you have been putting in and the reward.

We have no control over so many events and we can't control how things will turn out in any given moment. What we do have, however, is control over the effort we make and the attitude we take. Nobody enjoys feeling like a failure, so if you see an experience as *you* having failed, you are far more likely to want to give up.

Instead, evaluate the effort you have made and focus on the lessons you have learnt – perhaps the time isn't right just yet. Deep in your heart, know that if you keep applying a consistent effort, your success is just around the corner!

Trish's story

The owner of a company that sold specialised software programs. Trish was an incredibly hard-working and disciplined woman who took to goal-setting like a duck to water. She created a vision for the future of her business, then set about designing short-, medium- and long-term goals. She remembered to make regular progress reviews of her goals and found that she was entirely on track, except for her financial targets.

Trish had improved her systems and processes, customer service and staff management. She had refined her target market and assessed all her marketing material. As far as she could see, she was achieving all her goals except the one that mattered – the numbers on the bottom line. When I spoke with her she was at her wits' end – she couldn't work out where she was going wrong. I talked with her about the timing difference between effort and reward. Initially she wasn't convinced. I explained how

(continued)

important it was not to give up, and to keep up the excellent efforts she had been making to date.

I encouraged her to review her goals and see what lessons she could learn for the future, but at no time was she to consider not achieving her financial goals as a failure.

Trish continued to work hard and, over time, she saw her sales figures pick up. The increase was slow at first but then sales began to increase dramatically. Because she had done so much behind-the-scenes work in her business, she was in the perfect position to capitalise on this growth. At the end of the next quarter, Trish confirmed that she had achieved more in sales that quarter than she had over the previous four quarters combined. And she had totally blitzed her financial goals.

Exercise

Success isn't always instant. Sometimes we have to work far longer and harder for it than we may have initially anticipated.

Quite often, when you feel like giving up, you discover that success is just around the corner. On the other hand, if you do give up you will never know how close to your dream you really were.

Make a note in your journal of three times in your life when you felt like giving up and didn't. Did your success eventually come? How did you feel when you finally achieved your goal? What did you learn from this experience?

You might also like to use some examples of other people you know, as well as people in the public eye who have overcome the odds to achieve their goals.

Look over any time you feel success is too far away, or you feel like giving up.

YOU HAVE LEARNT SO MUCH ALREADY

If you are to create a life you really love, one that is filled with *real* success and happiness, you can't just rely on learning a few new things. You need to commit to consistently applying everything you have learnt. This is never more important than when you're facing tough times and the road ahead seems paved with obstacles.

Take a moment to look at what you have learnt since you began reading this book and how you can apply the lessons in each chapter to overcoming obstacles and working through the tough times.

Rediscover your dreams – Chapter 1

When you began to discover your dreams, you opened yourself up to a world filled with new possibilities. You took the first step towards making those dreams a reality by writing them down and thinking about what your life would be like if you lived in a perfect world. You learnt to find ways to include your dreams in your current life, focused on the power of positivity and began to believe it might be possible to make some of those dreams a reality.

Make the time to stay in touch with your dreams. This is never more important than when you are going through tough times. Enjoy some quality quiet time each day. While you are dreaming about your future, take note of everything you value about your present.

No matter how difficult things are, don't forget to keep believing in the power of positivity. Believe that you have the power to create exactly the kind of life you dream about.

Stay true to what matters – Chapter 2

Understanding your values is the key to creating a life filled with *real* success and happiness. You know what is important to you and with that knowledge it will be much easier to make decisions.

When times are tough and obstacles block your path, it is crucial to stay true to the things that matter most to you. When you are not in alignment with your values everything will feel more difficult, as if you are going against your inner flow. Be honest about your values; no one value is more 'valuable' than another, so make sure you stay true to what is right for you.

Remember, as long as you live in alignment with your values, you are already on the way to living your best life.

Examine your beliefs and self-talk – Chapter 3

When things aren't going to plan, don't blame the world for your lack of progress. Instead, look inside and ask yourself, How do I hold myself back? You will quickly find that if you adopt a positive perspective, things won't seem as bad as they once did.

Don't spend time criticising your efforts, instead congratulate yourself for getting as far as you have. During tough times it's important to identify and eliminate any limiting beliefs. Take an objective view, reframe your thoughts and use powerful affirmations to reform your thinking.

Make sure you are not creating obstacles by engaging in limiting or self-sabotaging behaviour. Stay positive and remember, if you believe it, you can achieve it!

If you believe it, you can achieve it!

Embrace your vision – Chapter 4

When things feel difficult, remember that you have taken ownership over the direction of your life and even if it doesn't feel like it right now, you are working towards making your vision for your future a reality.

Use the vivid visual and mental images of your vision to re-inspire and motivate yourself to keep going. You know exactly what direction you want for your life. Don't let temporary obstacles or setbacks send you off course.

Bring your future a little closer to your present with simple, inexpensive things you can do to make your dream life feel more like a reality.

Ensure your goals are realistic and attractive – Chapter 5

If it's been a while since you've reviewed your goals, now is the time to make sure they have remained SMART – Specific, Measurable, Achievable, Realistic and Time-based. You may have created what you believed were SMART goals, only to find that when you start on them, they aren't as realistic as you thought.

Don't fall into the trap of using negative language when thinking or speaking about your goals. Make sure you always represent your goals as positive, present tense and deeply personal statements.

When you experience tough times, identify two or three quick wins or short-terms goals that will help you to maintain your sense of progress.

No matter how far away your goals might seem, never give up, never give up, never give up!

Buff up your confidence – Chapter 6

It is important not to let obstacles or setbacks affect your self-confidence. Believe in yourself because of who you are, not just what you are capable of achieving.

Have you fallen into the trap of being an over-achiever, always trying to do too much, striving for perfection and worrying that nothing you do will ever be good enough? Remember, life is an experience, not a competition, so don't compare your progress against that of anyone else. As long as you have given your best, it will always be good enough.

If you are feeling discouraged or disillusioned, review your list of all your positive qualities and take the time to acknowledge how special you really are.

Don't be afraid to revise your plan – Chapter 7

Having a plan increases your chances of getting to where you want to go in the shortest possible time and with the fewest deviations. However, it is important to remember that your plan is simply your best estimation or educated guess at a given point in time.

As you work on your plan you might find you need to revise some of the deadlines or rearrange the order in which you need to complete various activities. Your plan is a work in progress – update it regularly to keep it relevant and realistic.

When you feel like things are off-track, remember the power of the perfect Monday. Set yourself up for a successful week by focusing on having the best Monday possible.

Review your resources – Chapter 8

Work with time, not against it! Overestimate how long you think it might take to overcome or work around your obstacles. Take the time to prioritise what needs to be done.

If you are feeling swamped and have no spare time, look at all the items on your to-do list and see where you can spend money to buy some time. If, on the other hand, you feel things are not moving fast enough, try to invest some additional time to take you closer to your goals.

Look at your support team of family, friends and experts and work out who can give you the support you need to overcome your current hurdles.

No matter how difficult things may seem, don't fall into bad habits. Eat well, drink water, exercise regularly and get enough sleep. Remember if you don't take care of yourself, the tough times will be even tougher!

Support your staying power – Chapter 9

Don't allow tough times to be an excuse for giving up. Adopt a mindset in which you can achieve anything you set out to do.

Make sure you are working on the right goals for you. If you find yourself working towards 'coulda', 'shoulda', or 'woulda' goals your subconscious will create all manner of obstacles to keep you from achieving something that isn't meaningful to you.

Set yourself up for success, not failure, by making sure that your goals are achievable. Check that your obstacles are not the result of overly ambitious or unrealistic objectives.

Identify any new habits you need to develop to help you stay committed during difficult times and find a structure that will keep you accountable for your progress.

Face your fears and carry on regardless – Chapter 10

Fear doesn't have to hold you back – it is the power you give your fears that holds you back. Never allow your fears to become an excuse for not achieving your goal.

There really is no such thing as failure; as long as you have given your best, you will always be a success. Accept that newfound success can be daunting and have confidence that you will be able to manage all the challenges it will bring.

Don't use obstacles to validate your fear that you don't deserve success or that it could all disappear at a moment's notice. Obstacles and tough times are not personal, they are a fact of life.

No matter how difficult things may become, never make your decisions from a place of fear. Remember to reframe your thoughts, reform your thinking and take action!

Exercise

Make a note in your journal of at least three things you have learnt from each of the chapters in this book. Take the time to write in detail and describe how you plan to continue applying those lessons on an ongoing basis in your life.

LIFE ISN'T ALWAYS EASY – BUT IT IS ALWAYS WORTH IT!

Creating the life of your dreams won't always be easy, but the results you achieve will always be worth it. It's important to keep your perspective as obstacles and tough times come your way. Although they might seem all-consuming or insurmountable at the time, in hindsight they won't seem nearly so critical.

> Creating the life of your dreams won't always be easy, but the results you achieve will always be worth it.

KEY LESSONS – WORKING THROUGH THE TOUGH TIMES

1. Don't let a 'but' get in the way of your future – 'buts' are nothing more than excuses, so overcome your limiting beliefs, build unshakeable self-confidence, face your fears and carry on regardless!

2. Things are either within your control or beyond your control. If they are beyond your control, learn to accept them. If they are within your control, do something about them.

3. Don't fall for intellectual illusions. Sometimes you can make things harder than they need to be as a way of protecting yourself from failure.

4. Learn to ask for all the help you need. Make sure you know who to call on for emotional, technical or logistical support.

5. It's OK to feel a little sorry for yourself – for a minute! If you want to take time out to lick your wounds, put a time limit on your 'pity party'.

6. Every experience in life gives you the chance to learn something. Look for the lesson and you will gain a positive outcome from any situation.

7. Sometimes there is a timing difference between effort and reward. Just because you are not where you wanted to be at this point in time, it doesn't mean you won't get there. Success is just around the corner.

8. Apply what you have learnt and remember it isn't always easy, but it is always worth it!

CHAPTER 12
Celebrating your success

Celebrating success is definitely one of my favourite topics. After all, what's the point of all the hard work you've done, if you don't acknowledge your progress!

All too often, people make the mistake of achieving one goal and starting work on the next without taking the time to recognise what they have achieved so far. Alternatively, they achieve a great result but are so intent on making every opportunity a learning experience that they direct all their attention to what they should do differently next time instead of taking the time to appreciate what they have done well this time.

Another mistake people make is celebrating only the big or master goal they have been working towards and not the smaller victories along the way. Celebrating all your successes acknowledges your efforts, builds your confidence and self-esteem and ultimately makes it all worthwhile!

IT'S A GOOD THING!

When we are young, many of us are encouraged not to brag, boast or anything else that can be seen as big-noting. And it's true, behaving like this can be very unattractive.

Bragging or boasting is about comparing yourself to others. It's about saying I have more than you. I'm better, smarter or richer than you. Comparing yourself to other people is not constructive. Even if you are sure that you are the smartest, richest or best, it's only a matter of time before someone else comes along and knocks off your crown.

Very few people can comfortably and confidently acknowledge their efforts because they are trying too hard to avoid bragging. Celebrating *your* success is acknowledging that you have been the very best you can be. It is not comparing yourself to others or celebrating a win at someone else's expense.

When you are positive and enthusiastic about your progress towards your goals, it can be exciting for people around you. They are inspired to believe that they, too, could succeed at working towards a new goal.

If you still feel shy about your success, don't worry. You don't *have* to involve anyone else at all. You can celebrate your success quietly and privately, just by taking a moment to acknowledge how hard you have worked and how far you have come.

CELEBRATE SUCCESSES, BIG AND SMALL

It is important to find opportunities for celebration in everything you do rather than saving it for the achievement of your major goals. Every goal is made up of a series of tasks and activities – you won't be able to achieve your goal unless you have diligently completed the majority of these steps. Take a positive approach by setting celebration points along the way.

Don't worry, you don't need to crack open a bottle of French Champagne, buy an expensive piece of jewellery or go on a world trip every time you acknowledge your success! The point of celebrating smaller successes is not to break the bank or blow your budget, it is to inspire you and keep you motivated while you work toward your long-term goals.

Look back over your plan and pay attention to all the significant steps you will need to take along the way, not just the key milestones or major goals. If your goal is to change career, you might want to acknowledge revising and updating your CV, the first informal meeting to discuss your new direction and your first interview. If your goal is to lose a significant amount of weight, acknowledgment points to consider might be successfully completing your food diary every day for a week, sticking to all your exercise goals for a week and losing your first 2 kilograms. Acknowledge that each of these steps will have made a critical contribution to your long-term goal.

If your goal is to start a new business venture you might want to celebrate completing the first draft of your business plan, your first meeting with your bank manager, the printing of your new business cards and signing the lease for your new premises.

These examples are not meant to be prescriptive, they are simply to highlight how many small milestones contribute to your success and why they are so important to your end goal.

ENJOY THE JOURNEY

Life is a journey, not a destination, as the expression goes, but it can be easy to forget this when you are head down, tail up, working towards your goal. You can become so focused on the end result that you lose sight of the pleasures along the way. Identifying success points on the way to your destination will make the entire experience of working towards your goal much more rewarding.

It take effort to make significant changes in your relationships, finances, health, fitness, career or any other area of your life. Sometimes making that effort will be easy; other times it can feel like your dreams are a long way off.

Celebrating your smaller successes heightens your awareness of the progress you're making towards your goal. You will feel that your goal is in sight, not out of reach forever.

CELEBRATE THE THINGS WITHIN YOUR CONTROL

Goal-setting is about focusing on what you want and when you want it. But so many events can influence your plan and it is a fact of life that some of these will be beyond your control. It is important not to let these external factors leave you with a sense of failure – as long as you have given your best, you will always be a success!

If you are looking for a new job, don't wait to get it before you celebrate. Instead, celebrate each time you come out of a job interview knowing that you couldn't have been better and there's nothing you could have done differently. After all, you can't make somebody select you for a job, but you can ensure that you have given yourself the best chance of selection.

If you are involved in competitive sport, don't just celebrate when you win or beat someone else, celebrate when you beat your personal best. You have no control over the efforts the other competitors make – who is having an off-day and who is in their prime. What you *can* control is the efforts you have made in your training sessions and the positive mindset you have on the day.

So many businesspeople only ever celebrate their success when they achieve financial goals. But financial outcomes, as important as they are, are just one way of measuring your progress. If your business goal is to achieve a certain turnover, there are many external factors that could influence that outcome – the financial position of your key clients, market conditions and the general economic climate. Any one of these factors could prevent you from achieving your financial target. Does that mean you have failed? Definitely not. Instead, look at all the work you have done behind the scenes as you worked towards this goal. You might have enhanced your sales process and your proposal documents. You might have increased the skills of your staff, or improved your systems and processes in anticipation of your bigger workload.

Each of these achievements are successes well worth celebrating, as they are significant developments in the long-term success of your business. When the external factors resolve themselves, you will be so much closer to your target because of the work you have already done.

Look at your goals and your plan and identify all the outcomes that are 100 per cent within your control versus those dependant on external factors. Make a point of celebrating when you achieve all your goals, especially those that are 100 per cent within your control.

Exercise

Think about something you wanted to achieve but weren't able to, for reasons that really were beyond your control. Maybe you wanted a particular job or promotion or perhaps you were competing for something, but you were pipped at the post. Take a moment to look back over the entire experience and identify two or three significant achievements that you could have celebrated along the way.

- How did you feel when you didn't achieve your goal?
- How would you have felt if you had taken the time to acknowledge some of the achievements you made on the way to your goal?
- What can you learn from this experience?

THE MORE SUCCESSFUL YOU FEEL, THE MORE SUCCESSFUL YOU WILL BECOME

Each time you celebrate your success, you are sending your subconscious a powerful message: I am a successful person! I am the kind of person who regularly experiences success.

The more successful you feel, the more successful you will become. You have already learnt that your subconscious mind accepts every piece of information it receives as fact. It never judges and it is not capable of evaluating the information it is given.

When you celebrate one of your smaller successes, one of the stepping stones on your journey, your subconscious doesn't say, 'Well, that was only a little goal, so you are only a little bit successful.' The only message your subconscious receives is that you have done something worth celebrating and therefore you must *be* successful!

Once your subconscious mind has received a loud and clear message about how successful you are, it does everything within its power to maintain this situation. Just as your subconscious mind accepts any limiting beliefs or negative self-talk as fact, then works towards perpetuating that reality, it follows exactly the same process with positive self-talk and empowering self-belief.

Many people are uncomfortable with the idea of celebrating their success, especially the smaller successes. The most common reason is a lack of self-worth or low self-esteem. If you feel deep down that you are not truly deserving of success, celebrating it will be in direct conflict with your negative self-belief.

You might be saying to yourself, 'I'll wait until I achieve the really big goal before I celebrate my progress,' but check if you are following that statement with 'if I ever get there!'

If your self-belief is not robust you will always question whether your efforts were good enough. You will never feel comfortable allowing yourself to feel proud of your efforts. You may find you are too busy criticising yourself, focusing on what you have done wrong or what you need to do differently next time, to take a moment to acknowledge what has gone well, here, in the present.

If you find yourself attributing your success to luck, even when you know you have worked hard, remind yourself – the harder you work, the luckier you get!

When I work hard and achieve my goals, I want to shout it from the rooftops, broadcast it on national television or sign-write it in the sky! Although I am usually more discreet than that, I feel confident that my success has been a direct result of the commitment and discipline I have applied and I am proud of those efforts.

I want to *believe* that I am a success. In fact, I enjoy affirming this belief whenever possible by celebrating all manner of accomplishments. Not every celebration is something I shout out loud about. Many are quiet, private celebrations, in which the party is in my heart. But trust me, I'm celebrating!

If you want to be successful you need to feel successful. Celebrating your success is an investment in your future, not just in the goals you are currently working on. If you create a mindset that supports success and *believe* you are a success, you will find it easy to continue to achieve all your goals.

**The more successful you feel,
the more successful you will become.**

Exercise

How do you feel about success? Do you believe you truly deserve it? Are you excited about the opportunity to celebrate your successes, big and small? Or do you find yourself cringing at the idea of acknowledging your efforts? Instead, do you focus on all the things you could improve and all the reasons why you shouldn't be celebrating?

Make a note in your journal describing your feelings about the recognition and celebration of success. If you find you are less than comfortable with the idea of acknowledging and celebrating your progress, create two or three powerful affirmations to reform these feelings. You might want to try:

- 'I always give 100 per cent and I deserve to celebrate my success!'
- 'I am comfortable and confident with success.'
- 'I am excited by opportunities to celebrate my success.'

SUCCESS IS CONTAGIOUS

One of the most positive aspects of success is that it's contagious – celebrating your success is the best way to spread it around! When people see that you have been successful, that you have been able to achieve your goals and change your life for the better, they can feel inspired to achieve their goals too. As discussed in Chapter 10, occasionally you might find that people resent your success. Don't let this put you off. It is most definitely about them, not you. Seeing you achieve your dreams makes them wonder why they are not achieving their own dreams, why they are still stuck in a rut, or living a life that is no longer fulfilling or rewarding. Rather than using this trigger as an opportunity to look within and do a bit of soul-searching, a chance to discover what they would like to change about their life and how they might go about doing it, these people direct their frustration at the source of their new thoughts – you!

While this experience may not be pleasant, don't try to change their life for them. Just be patient and recognise that your success has upset their status quo. Regardless of what they say or how they behave, remember that their anger is only with themselves.

The good news is that nearly everyone you know will be pleased for you. Every time you celebrate your success, not only will you build your own confidence and increase your self-esteem, you automatically excite and inspire the people around you.

THE ART OF REWARDING YOURSELF

If celebrating my success is one of my favourite pastimes, rewarding myself is definitely high on my list too! Most people associate rewarding themselves with spending money. Although a shopping trip can certainly be pleasurable, you can also reward yourself with time, space or experiences. An afternoon in the park or a walk along the beach can be just as special as a new outfit, a night on the town or a holiday somewhere special.

If you do have enough money, don't be afraid to spend a little on treating yourself. Celebrate your success with the purchase of something you have been dreaming about, a special bottle of wine, a night at the theatre, or a weekend away.

So many people feel they can't spend their money on themselves, regardless of how much they have. They are trapped in a poverty consciousness, in which they feel every spare cent should be saved, invested, put into the mortgage or squirreled away in some other fashion. Whilst it's important to provision for your future, I believe that you need to live for today. Spending a little money on yourself is a different kind of investment. It's an investment in your self-esteem – you are sending yourself a clear message that says, 'I'm worth it!'

If your goal is to save money or if you simply don't have much to spare, you will need to find other, more creative ways of celebrating your success. Rewarding yourself for your progress can come in many forms and while it can be lovely to buy yourself treats, a quality reward doesn't have to cost you anything.

When I first started my business, I put every cent I made back into the business as an investment in my long-term success. But I didn't stop rewarding myself. I remembered all the inexpensive ways I used to reward myself back when I was a student or first working. Buying a book rather than borrowing it from the library was a treat. Taking a long lunch and lingering over a favourite magazine was a luxury. When I did experience financial success, I spent a little money on a reward for myself, but when my successes were of a different kind, I found other ways to reward myself.

Jenny's story

The owner of a successful event management company, Jenny had built her business from scratch and now it had an annual turnover of several million dollars. Although she knew she had worked hard to build her business, she had never really taken the time to acknowledge how much she had achieved – she was too busy moving from one goal to the next.

She came to coaching to further develop her management and leadership skills. The idea of creating a positive team culture was important to her and we discussed the value of recognition and reward when motivating others. Jenny confessed that she found it difficult to know when and how to reward her team members – it just didn't come naturally to her.

I wasn't surprised. It's hard to reward others when you're not comfortable rewarding yourself, so I asked Jenny to make a list of at least 20 things she had achieved since she had started her business.

She found she actually began to enjoy acknowledging all of her achievements. Once her list was complete, I asked her to identify a way of rewarding herself for each of her achievements and to commit to giving herself these rewards over the next six months.

(continued)

The only condition was that while the rewards didn't need to be expensive, they did have to be of value to her.

After a hesitant start, Jenny got into the habit of rewarding herself. She spent afternoons in the garden, went to the movies during the day and had coffee and croissants in bed with the Sunday papers — things she would never normally do. She even bought an artwork for her office wall — she told me she just knew she deserved it!

Once Jenny became comfortable with rewarding herself, she became a natural at rewarding others. She found it easy to identify when her staff had given their best and knew instinctively what rewards would be of most value to them. The more Jenny recognised her team's success, the more effort they each put into being successful, and her business went from strength to strength.

Exercise

Look at your list of goals once more and think about how you are going to reward yourself for each of your achievements. Make a list of things you have been looking forward to buying, doing, seeing or experiencing. Remember, your rewards don't have to cost you anything. A lie-in with your favourite book can be just as rewarding as a big night out at an expensive restaurant.

Your rewards don't *all* need to be pre-planned though, you can have plenty of fun rewarding yourself spontaneously too!

The most important thing to remember is that rewarding yourself mustn't compromise or conflict with the goals you are working to achieve. Don't reward your weight-loss achievements with a feast of your favourite indulgences, or your savings progress with a big shopping trip! Make sure that the reward you choose is a celebration, not a setback.

ACKNOWLEDGE *REAL* SUCCESS

I began this book by discussing the importance of achieving *real* success and discovering what in this world matters most to you. So many people tell me they haven't achieved anything noteworthy lately, simply because they are not working on big-money, big-impact or major-change goals.

Remember that one of the most important goals you will ever set is being the best you can be. Any time you have given 100 per cent to what you have chosen to do, you *are* being the best you can be, and that is the ultimate success.

Any time you find yourself striving to achieve what someone else has achieved or wanting to keep up with your friends, colleagues or other family members, *stop!* You are wasting your time. Sure a bigger house, faster car or better job might seem like something you want, it might even feel good for a while, but unless the house, car or job is a meaningful goal for you, it won't bring you pleasure for long. If you pursue this path, too often you will find yourself having worked extremely hard only to question what it was all for.

Success can be found in doing anything you choose to do, well. There is enormous success in being a good parent, a loving partner or a trusted friend. Success can be as simple as feeding your family healthy meals each night while sticking to a budget, or staying calm and not lowering yourself to the petty battles of office politics.

Success might be maintaining a faithful marriage no matter how many times you have been tempted to stray. It could be taking time out from work to care for a loved one or making the decision to take better care of yourself.

When you strive for success that someone else has defined for you, be that your parents, your peer group or the powerful influence of the media, your experience of success will be empty and short-lived. When you achieve your own, deeply personal goals, no matter how large or small they might be, this experience of success will truly enrich your life.

Brendan's story

Ever since he was a small child, Brendan had wanted to be a multimillionaire. His mantra was '40 million by 40' and at 36 he had made a solid start on his goal with several successful property ventures.

All of his goals were about making money or spending money. There were goals about deal size and profit margins, and goals for the big house on the harbour and the new sports car he wanted to buy.

He came to coaching because he was feeling frustrated with his progress over the past 12 months. Although the property market had generally been poor, Brendan wanted to know what he should be doing differently from a self-management point of view to increase his chances of success. He wondered if he needed to become more strategic, better organised, more

(continued)

efficient or clearer in his delegation. The one thing he was sure he didn't need to improve was his ability to set goals.

I asked Brendan what mattered most to him outside of work and, being the father of two little girls, he immediately said 'Family'. I asked him what else was important, and he added 'My relationship with my wife and my strength and fitness'.

Although I was happy to work with Brendan on his professional performance, I explained that if he wanted to experience *real* success and happiness, he needed to focus on bringing success into all the areas of his life that were important to him, not just work and finance. At first he didn't know where to begin, but with a little coaching he was able to set goals that included increasing the amount of time he spent with his daughters, romantic dinners and weekend breaks with his wife, and several weekly sessions with his fitness trainer.

Within a short time Brendan was feeling much happier. Although he was still feeling frustrated by the state of the market, he had realised that this wasn't the only important thing in his life. The increased enjoyment he was feeling by focusing some of his energy on other things that mattered was more than making up for it!

Exercise

Think about all the goals you have set. Do a quick double-check and make sure that everything you are working towards really matters to you. Check that nothing on your list is there for the wrong reason – for example, keeping up with others or fulfilling someone else's expectations for your life.

Make the decision to continue with all the work you have done in the exercises throughout this book. Look at your diary and set aside time each week to continue reviewing your goals and assessing your progress. Commit to applying everything you have learnt by being the best you can be, each and every day.

If you want your life to be filled with *real* success and happiness, you need to be willing to work for it – and this is your chance!

LIVE YOUR LIFE AS IF IT'S A CELEBRATION!

While celebrating your achievements and your progress is important, it's nowhere near as important as celebrating the fact you are alive, and that you are *living* your life.

Learn to live as though each experience is a lesson and each day is a blessing. See how many fulfilling experiences you can fall in love with and how much love you can fill your life with. Make the decision to continue applying all the lessons you have learnt from this book and make a commitment to create the very best life for yourself.

Learn to live as though each experience is a lesson and each day is a blessing.

KEY LESSONS – CELEBRATING YOUR SUCCESS

1. Celebrating your success isn't about bragging or boasting. It's about acknowledging your efforts and how far you have come.
2. Don't just celebrate the big achievements, celebrate the smaller ones along the way – each one is a significant contribution to your overall success.
3. Life is a journey, not a destination, so make sure you take the time to enjoy each step of the way.
4. You can't control all outcomes, but you can influence them with the efforts you make. Make sure you celebrate the part of your goal that is within your control.
5. The more successful you feel, the more successful you will become. Celebrating your success today is an investment in the future.
6. When you achieve your goals you can inspire the people around you to achieve their goals, too. Success is contagious – spread yours around!
7. When you reward yourself for your success, you send a very clear message to your subconscious that says – I'm worth it!
8. *Real* success is simply being the best you can be and achieving the things in life that matter most to you.

Author's Note

Finishing this book is not the end – it's just the beginning!

You have made a significant investment by taking the time to read this book and complete the exercises, but we both know the real challenge was never simply finishing this book; it is taking all the things that you have learnt and all the answers you have discovered and applying them to your life. Now it's time to make your investment pay off by turning your dreams into reality.

As you work towards creating your very best life, you will find it useful to refer back to individual chapters and to my website www.domoniquebertolucci. com/yourbestlife for extra support. You will also find that even though you have completed the exercises once, doing them again at different times in your life will be valuable, especially when you are facing a particular challenge, your circumstances have changed, or you simply feel you need a refresher.

Don't let this book get dusty! Keep it close to hand and refer back to it as often as you need to keep yourself motivated and feeling positive, as you create the life of your dreams.

You only have one life – it's important that you really LOVE it!

With love and best wishes,

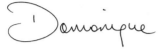

PS: I would love to hear how your journey is progressing and how reading this book has impacted on your life. Of course, I also love to hear a good success story! You can write to me at domonique@domoniquebertolucci.com

Acknowledgments

There are so many people whose support I need to acknowledge. My first thanks go to my agent Tara Wynne and commissioning editor Vanessa Radnidge for believing in *Your Best Life* as much as I do.

Thank you to Lisa Highton and all the team at Hachette Australia who continue to surpass my expectations. To Ellie Exarchos for your beautiful cover and to Joanna Dye, photographer and friend, for capturing exactly what I was looking for – a picture of the *real* me…on a *really* good day!

Thanks to branding guru and great friend Brooke Alexander for sharing my vision and helping me to turn it into www.domoniquebertolucci.com

There are people in your life who help to define it and I would like to thank these special girls who knew me before I knew myself: Adele, Brigette, Callie, Deanne, Fiona, Jane, Liz, Mary, Sarah and Sophie. To Lisa, for love and friendship; with special thanks to Alecia for so many things, especially the suggestion that my ideas should be 'bottled', which led to the birth of this book; and to Tristan, who has always believed in my dreams as if they were her own.

To each of my clients, thank you for inviting me to be a part of your journey. It is a privilege, and I am honoured to have learnt so much from you.

Thank you to my wonderful family – Mum and Dad, my brother Jeff – for unconditional love, endless support and sharing my excitement as this book became a reality. An extra special thank you to Mum, who spent countless hours proofreading the first draft.

Finally, my biggest thanks go to my husband, Paul, for everything, always.

Domonique Bertolucci is widely recognised as an expert on how to achieve *real* success. She has spent hundreds of hours coaching high-achieving business owners and executives — people who want to achieve ambitious professional goals, without burning out or losing sight of who they are and why they wanted it in the first place.

Highly sought after as a keynote speaker, Domonique gets audiences thinking about what it is they *really* want from life and why they haven't been living that way up until now. Her presentations leave people feeling motivated, inspired, and with a very strong desire to take the actions they need to start making it happen.

Born and raised in Perth, Domonique's first career as a fashion model took her to London at 22. There she underwent a dramatic transformation — from model to corporate high-flyer. After ten years in the fiercely competitive and cut-throat world of investment banking, where she earned a reputation for turning around dysfunctional and under-achieving teams, and managing high performers, Domonique decided to return to Australia.

On her return she established Success Strategies, a company that delivers personal and professional development programs to organisations that are serious about investing in their most important asset — their people. Success Strategies offers a range of coaching programs as well as the Unlimited Ambition™ workshop series. A new workshop, *Your Best Life*, has recently been introduced as a companion program to this book.

Domonique is an ambassador for Opportunity International, the microfinance organisation. A percentage of the royalties from this book will be donated to Opportunity International and used to establish a Trust Bank, which will provide loans to poor entrepreneurs in developing countries.

Domonique regularly appears on television and in the print media. She lives in Sydney with her husband, and in her spare time can be found at the cinema, practising yoga and keeping up the great Italian tradition of feeding the people you love.

Your Best Life is her first book.

To find out more about Domonique Bertolucci or Success Strategies programs, please visit www.domoniquebertolucci.com or www.success-strategies.com.au or call 1300 137 304 (Aust) or +612 9232 2440 (intl).

Domonique has created a special area on her website just for readers of *Your Best Life*. Log onto *www.domoniquebertolucci.com/yourbestlife* for a range of free resources, including worksheets, tools templates and extra tips, all designed to give you extra support as you begin to create the life of your dreams. The members area also contains twelve 30-minute audio recordings to support you as you complete each chapter*.

You will also find other resources on Domonique's website. *LOVE your LIFE* is a free monthly e-zine overflowing with inspiration and motivation. Each issue contains tips, interviews, articles and book reviews to help you get the most out of your life. *LOVE your LIFE* is published on the first Wednesday of each month. Visit *www.domoniquebertolucci.com* to subscribe.

You may also like to access *Success Strategies: at work*, a free monthly newsletter that focuses on leadership strategies and professional performance tips for executives and business owners. *Success Strategies: at work* is published on the third Wednesday of each month. Visit *www.success-strategies.com.au* to subscribe.

---

* A fee applies to the audio program